AR in Surgery: Planning the Future

Shireen

First Printing, 2024

Table of Contents

Chapter 1: Introduction

1.1 Rationale

Surgeons are often early adopters of technologies that improve surgical experiences (Khor et al., 2016). During image-guided surgery (IGS) surgeons are required to integrate multi-modal imaging data from several sources while performing the procedure on the patient. Frequent switching between the two-dimensional (2D) monitors and the surgical site places a heavy cognitive load on the surgeon. Figure 1.1 shows a recently observed operating room at Groote Schuur hospital in Cape Town, South Africa. The surgical setup, which includes images from multiple modalities, demonstrates the need for reducing the cognitive load that surgeons experience during image-guided interventions. This setup is similar to that described in (Sielhorst, 2008) fo minimally invasive spine surgery.

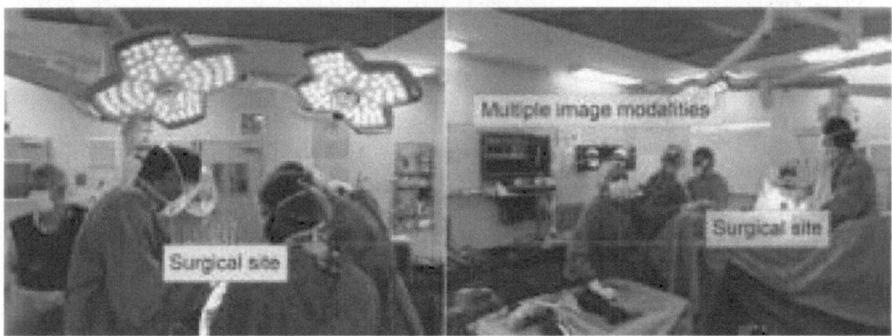

Figure 1.1: Example of image-guided intervention in an operating room at Groote Schuur Hospital (2018). As shown by the arrows the surgeon is required to look away from the surgical site to integrate multi-modal imaging data from several sources whilst performing the intervention on the patient.

In addition to surgeons, radiologists and clinicians also experience information overload as a result of the vast improvement in image spatial resolution and image display capabilities (Ferroli et al., 2013). Various modalities and techniques have been established since an X-ray was first used in a surgical operation by John Hall Edwards in 1896. These include 2D images such as ultrasound and fluoroscopic X-ray as well as three-dimensional (3D) volume modalities such as computed tomography (CT) and magnetic resonance imaging (MRI). 2D images and 3D image volumes are termed anatomical imaging. Functional imaging modalities include positron emission tomography (PET), optical imaging, electroencephalogram (EEG) and magnetoencephalogram (MEG). The combination of anatomical and functional imaging, such as in functional MRI (fMRI) or single-photon emission computed tomography (SPECT/CT), has allowed clinicians to understand physiological aspects of the human anatomy which is critical during IGS (Paul et al., 2005).

Recent advances in computer-mediated reality technologies have created a shift in the way clinicians may be able to interact with the aforementioned image modalities (Rodrigues et al., 2017). Milgram and Kishino (1994) created a taxonomy for these immersive technologies, the reality-virtuality (RV) continuum. This continuum encompasses environments ranging from the completely physical world to the completely virtual world. Real environments are our normal state, but as soon as computer-generated data is added to enhance the senses this becomes a mixed reality (MR) experience. Mixed reality is considered as the space between the real and the virtual, encompassing both augmented reality (AR) and augmented virtuality (AV). In AR, the virtual augments the real; whereas, in AV, the real augments the virtual. Virtual reality (VR) is at the far end of the RV spectrum with the user completely transported into a virtual environment. Computer-mediated reality is the umbrella term for both MR and VR technology.

Augmented reality combines human experience and intuition with the computational power of computers; research has shown that making use of AR Head Mounted Display (HMD) systems have the potential to address the cognitive load experienced during surgery through implementing a holographic view of patient data in situ (Vávra et al., 2017). Using an AR HMD system, holographic anatomical structures of the patient's blood vessels, nerves, and bones can be seamlessly juxtaposed in the field of view (FOV) of the surgeon in situ (Pratt et al., 2018). Navigating the volumetric data through AR 3D user interfaces instead of a 2D computer monitor has also been found to be more natural for clinicians to analyse the spatial, anatomical, and functional features for surgical planning (Eck et al., 2016). However, developing computer-mediated reality systems presents complex software and hardware engineering challenges due to the diverse range of technologies required to implement solutions that do not over encumber the user (Rodrigues et al., 2017). In the past, the complexity of developing an AR HMD system required prohibitive time and resources for the design and development of prototypes to give the impression of a holographic user interface. However, with the release of commercial AR HMD products like the Microsoft HoloLens (Figure 1.2), the technology has been made more accessible (Rodrigues et al., 2017).

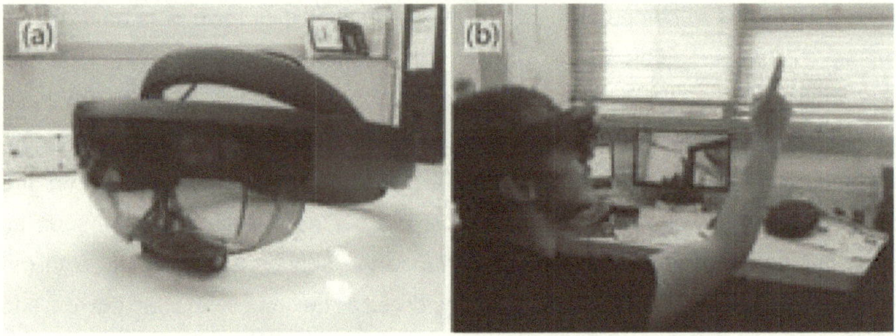

Figure 1.2: The Microsoft HoloLens. (a) A front-on view of the Microsoft HoloLens. (b) Author wearing the Microsoft HoloLens, the virtual object being viewed is seen on the computer screen in the background.

The utility of an AR HMD system during surgery is that the imagery for procedural guidance can be displayed as a holographic image on the surgical site as opposed to the current visualization techniques which rely on multiple 2D displays. Nevertheless, the patient-specific data (the virtual objects) must be registered accurately to aid the procedure; failing this, the clinician could be misled and cause serious harm to the patient. The motivation for this project was to gain an understanding of computer-mediated reality systems for medicine and to use that understanding to design and develop an AR HMD system for use in medicine. Such a system is henceforth referred to as an AR HMD medical system.

1.2 Aim and objectives

This project was an exemplar for the utility of computer-mediated reality technology in aiding pre-surgical planning, intra-operative guidance, post-surgical assessment, and rehabilitation progress tracking. The aim of this project was to develop and demonstrate the use of an AR HMD medical system. Image-guided surgery of the hand and wrist was selected as the IGS procedure to explore the development of an AR HMD medical system as this anatomy exemplified the complexities of creating a 3D volume as a virtual object to be visualized.

The objectives were as follows:

1. Developing system specifications of an AR HMD medical system for the reconstruction, registration, and visualisation of 3D patient-specific image scans specifically for surgery and broader clinical applications.
2. Applying the AR HMD medical system by registering the computer-generated AR view of a 3D hand and bone geometry onto a surgical site in situ.

1.3 Scope of work

For the project, the surgical site was defined as a 3D printed version of hand and bone virtual objects. One of the core functional requirements of an AR HMD medical systems is the accuracy in the registration of the virtual image to the real-world object. Registration accuracy, spatial registration, and spatial stability are critical to the success in the development of an AR HMD medical system. The hypothesis of this project was that it is feasible to create an AR HMD medical system to register a holographic view of a 3D geometry to a surgical site in situ using a commercially available AR HMD system, the Microsoft HoloLens. In combination with the Microsoft HoloLens, user calibration, fiducial marker, and markerless tracking were used as solutions for registering the virtual object to the surgical site.

Three prototype AR HMD systems were developed to validate the aforementioned registration techniques; i.e. 1) user calibrated -, 2) fiducial marker -, and 3) markerless tracking AR HMD systems. Quantitative analysis experiments were completed to assess the registration accuracy and spatial capabilities of the three developed AR HMD systems.

1.4 Ethical considerations

An application for ethics clearance was submitted and approved by the UCT Faculty of Health Sciences Ethics Committee to use imaging data for the development of a virtual object from a captured image modality data set HREC REF 458/2018.

1.5 Structure of the dissertation

The rest of this dissertation is structured as follows: chapter 2 presents a taxonomy for computer-mediated reality technology and describes a review of use cases for the technology in computer-assisted surgery. Chapter 3 presents the essential technical and technological requirements for creating AR HMD medical systems where virtual objects are registered to a specific location in the real-world environment.

From the literature, user calibration, fiducial marker, and markerless tracking have been reported as solutions for registration in combination with AR HMD medical systems. Chapter 4 describes the different sets of software development kits (SDKs), software settings, and hardware components required to achieve the corresponding registration method and virtual object visualization in the FOV via the selected AR HMD system. For the purpose of this dissertation, each registration solution is considered a separate stand-alone AR HMD system. This is because each registration's algorithmic pipeline contained some idiosyncratic components that were distinct from the others. Chapter 4 also details the materials selected to explore the development of the three AR HMD systems to assess the validity of the identified registration methods to align the virtual to the real.

The validation experiments to assess the three developed AR HMD systems are detailed in chapters 5, 6, and 7. Final discussion of the results and the future work required to realize an AR HMD medical system are presented in chapter 8.

Chapter 2: Review of computer-mediated realities in medicine

Kishino and Milgram (1994) created a taxonomy for computer-mediated reality technologies, the reality-virtuality continuum. Kersten-Oertel et al., (2012) defined a taxonomy to classify computer-mediated reality visualization techniques used in IGS based on the type of data, the type of visualization processing the data undergoes before being presented to the end-user, and the means of the view (display). The two taxonomies are combined in the following sections to classify the reality-virtuality continuum in terms of the display technology used. By combining the taxonomies, a framework to identify the state of the human-computer interaction during each step of the image-guided surgical process flow as defined by Beaulieu et al. (2008) has been created (Figure 2.1). This chapter also reviews the use of computer-mediated realities in medicine.

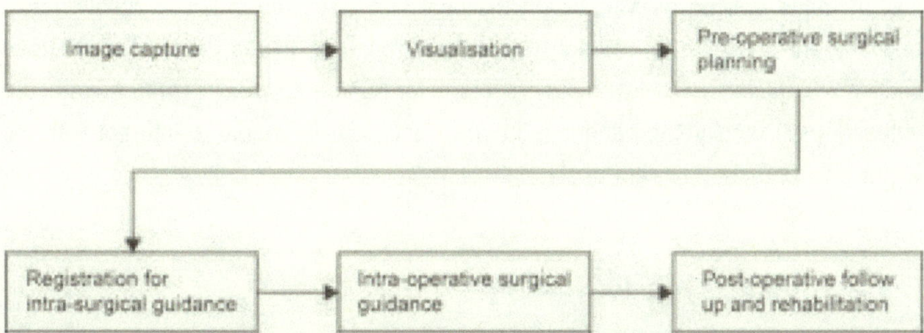

Figure 2.1: The cycle of care process flow for IGS, adapted from Beaulieu et al., (2008).

2.1 The reality-virtuality continuum

With image-guided surgery, the operating room, the medical personnel, the patient, the surgical table, the tools, and all monitors form part of the real environment. Virtual objects are defined as any digital representations or models of the real-world objects (Kersten-Oertel et al., 2012). To distinguish between real and virtual, it is important to note the degree of real-world knowledge, the quality of the visuals and the extent of how present the user feels in the displayed scene. The reality-virtuality continuum encompasses environments ranging from the completely real to the completely virtual. Real environments are our normal state; in a clinical setting, a real environment could be an operating room where the attending surgeon is completing the operation. A real environment can also be the viewing of a live video feed from an endoscope, multimodal images or X-ray images via a C-arm. When computer-generated data (virtual objects) is added to enhance any of these scenarios, this becomes a computer-mediated experience (Mann et al., 2018). Within the reality-virtuality framework, Milgram and Kishino (1994) defined three categories, Mixed reality (MR), Virtual reality (VR) and Tele-presence.

2.2 Mixed reality

An MR environment is one in which real and virtual objects are presented together within a single display. In other words, any experience that is between fully real and fully virtual is defined as MR. When the user is transported to a completely virtual environment and able to interact with the environment, this is defined as VR (see section 2.5). Mixed reality is the superset term for Augmented reality (AR), Augmented virtuality (AV), and VR experiences in which the user is unable to interact with the virtual environment (Milgram et al., 1994).

2.3 Augmented reality

Augmented reality interfaces are used to enhance interactions with real environments (Billinghurst et al., 2014). With AR the user is not transported out of their environment, but rather, using a display or projection, more information is added to the view of their environment. A medical example of AR is the VeinViewer Vision system, which uses infrared light and sensors to differentiate between the haemoglobin concentration in the bloodstreams and the surrounding tissue, subsequently mapping the veins onto the skin of the patient using projection (Kim et al., 2012). Azuma (1997) defined the widely accepted key functional requirements for a system to be classified as AR and Billinghurst et al. (2014) used the three functional characteristics established by

Azuma (1997) to create a set of technical requirements for an AR system. Both sets of requirements are detailed in Table 2.1.

Table 2.1: Azuma's (1997) functional requirements vs. Billinghurst et al.'s (2014) technical requirements of an AR system.

Nr.	Functional Requirement	Technical requirement
1.	Runs interactively and in real time.	Image processing to combine the interactive computer-generated (CG) graphics with the real-time view of the user and respond to the user's inputs.
2.	Registered in 3D and aligns the real and virtual objects.	A tracking system to track the FOV of the user to enable the virtual images to appear anchored in the real world.
3.	Combines real and virtual content in a real environment.	A display that can merge the real and virtual images.

Sielhorst et al., (2008) detailed several fundamental classes of AR display technology, including their specific limitations and advantages to clinicians for surgical guidance. A brief description of each type of display technology is presented below.

2.3.1 Monitor-based AR displays

Monitor-based AR is a non-immersive experience and uses handheld or physical display devices such as tablets or smartphones as windows to add more information to the real environment (Billinghurst et al., 2014). Examples of monitor-based AR display software applications are Visible bodies (https://www.visiblebody.com/ar) and smartphone and tablet AR applications for anatomy education by 3D4Medical's (https://3d4medical.com/) that allow the viewing of augmented anatomy content in real-world scenarios.

2.3.2 Stereoscopic AR display

Stereo vision, or stereoscopic vision, is the principle behind depth perception and it allows for 3D understanding through combining slightly different images from each eye (Solovey et al., 2015). Figure 2.2 shows the zSpace (https://zspace.com/), a semi-immersive interactive 3D stereoscopic display. The zSpace system consists of full colour, high-resolution stereoscopic display with embedded cameras for tracking, a pair of tracked circularly polarized glasses, and a six-degree-of-freedom (6-DOF) 3D stylus to allow for interaction with the virtual views (Mandalika et al., 2018). When interacting with the 3D holographic simulations, three perceptual abilities are leveraged, namely stereo vision, motion parallax and proprioception.

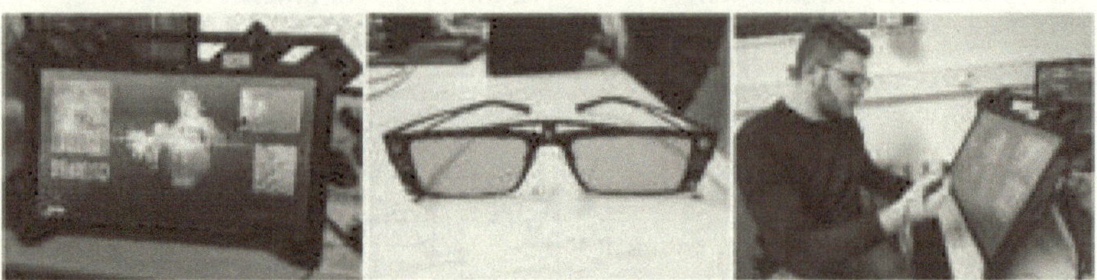

Figure 2.2: The zSpace system consists of a stereoscopic display, a pair of tracked circularly polarized glasses, and a 6-DOF 3D stylus.

2.3.3 Spatial AR displays

Spatial AR displays computer-generated data directly onto the physical objects and is often referred to as projection AR (Carmigniani et al., 2011). The image rendering source needs to stay in its position in 3D defined space, i.e. fixed spatially. The VeinViewer system mentioned earlier is an example of a spatial AR display. Spatial AR makes use of video projectors, optical elements or screens in combination with tracking technologies to display the computer-generated data directly onto the object being augmented (Chen et al., 2017).

Autostereoscopic image overlay systems display 3D stereoscopic images without the need for special eyeglasses. By combining autostereoscopic and integral videography, a 3D image can be superimposed onto the patient. A typical stereoscopic system comprises a special display with a convex microlens array bonded onto a liquid crystal panel and tracking technology. The holographic visualization is created by projecting light rays through the complex microlens array onto the tracked object being augmented (Ma et al., 2019).

2.3.4 Magic Mirrors

A subcategory of monitor-based and spatial AR displays is a system referred to as a Magic Mirror. A Magic Mirror refers to an AR system with a large digital display employing the mirror metaphor as the users see a reflection of themselves with virtual information superimposed on the display (Bork et al., 2019). An example of such a system is the Magic Mirror developed by Blum et al., (2012) for anatomy education. The system provides an AR in-situ visualization of anatomies such as 3D models of organs and skeletal views via a large display that "acts as a mirror". The virtual view mimics the tracked movement of the user measured via an RGB depth camera, the Microsoft Kinect (Kugelmann et al., 2018).

2.3.5 Heads-up-displays (HUD) or AR Windows

This display technology forms part of the Spatial AR display classification, however, the virtual image is projected onto half-silvered mirrors or an angled window, which is situated between the user and the real environment. The angle of the display reflects the virtual image into the optical path of the real image. Heads-up-displays are also referred to as spatial see-through displays as the screen and image projector module are fixed. An example of a HUD in medicine is an operating microscope enhanced with a semi-transparent mirror into the optics (Sielhorst et al., 2008). The AR HUD operating microscope could also be described as a see-through AR display. When a see-through display is mounted on the user's head, it becomes an AR head-mounted display (HMD) as discussed below.

2.3.6 Head-mounted AR displays

The concept of an AR HMD was first introduced by Ivan Sutherland who developed a system that used spectacles containing two miniature cathode-ray tubes to create the AR view (Sutherland, 1968). The HMD was worn to create an apparent holographic view in the FOV of the user. Modern optical see-through AR HMD use stereoscopy and optical see-through mirrors to reflect computer-generated images onto the user's eyes and create an augmented view. More simply put, it is a HUD mounted on the user's head. Besides standalone optical see-through AR HMD, there are numerous tethered solutions as well. An optical see-through HMD provides a real environment view and requires more advanced technologies to correctly place the holographic view in the environment due to changes in the user's head position/orientation. With AR visualization, spatial placement refers to the position a virtual object occupies in a predefined space in 3D.

A subcategory of HMD AR is video see-through HMD. These are created by combining video cameras and VR HMD systems. Recently, untethered video see-through HMDs have been developed through combining smartphones with headgear such as the Samsung Gear VR (www.samsung.com/global/galaxy/gear-vr/). The Samsung Gear VR (Figure 2.3) uses the video camera from the smartphone to capture the real-world view. The recorded footage of the real world is combined with the computer-generated images via the mobile device's display, with the two replaceable lenses in the headgear creating the stereoscopic effect.

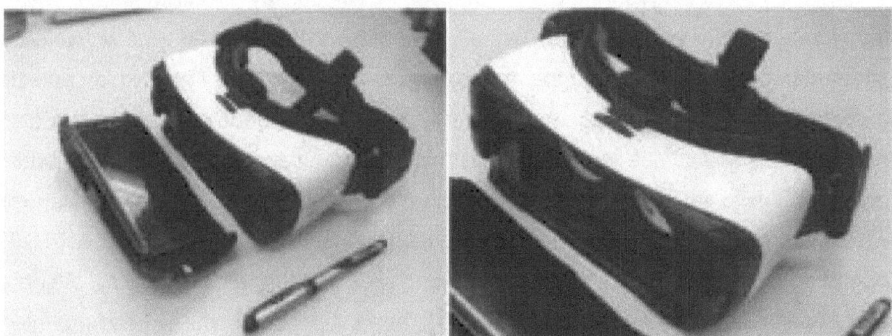

Figure 2.3: Samsung Gear VR, an example of a video see-through HMD.

Currently, the third type of HMD is the retinal projection display. With this type of display, the AR image is drawn onto the retina of the eye using a low-power laser beam. However, this see-through HMD is currently not as common as the optical see-through or video see-through HMD. Augmented reality HMD systems are well suited for IGS as they can be used without compromising the environment's sterility (Sielhorst et al., 2008).

2.4 Augmented virtuality

Real objects are physical entities that conform to the laws of physics and time. Augmented virtuality refers to real objects introduced into a virtual environment. The experience can be immersive or partially immersive (Kersten-Oertel et al., 2012). The user's knowledge of the real world is limited to the real-world objects presented in the completely synthetic environment, with the visual of the real-world object being photo-realistic. For example, by using Chroma key compositing (removing a real-world object from a coloured background, typically green), the user can see their hands in the virtual environment. Paul et al. (2005) developed an application that employed the principle of AV to merge an image of the visible brain surface captured during the surgery with the virtual anatomical and physiological models derived from the preoperative medical images on a display in the operating room.

2.5 Virtual reality

Virtual reality is at the far end of the spectrum and describes an experience whereby the user is completely immersed in a synthetic world and can interact with different elements in this virtual environment (Milgram & Kishino, 1994). With VR, the effectiveness of the virtual environments is characterised by the level of immersion the user experiences. In a fully immersive virtual environment, the user is unbound and can manipulate the virtual objects using an input device such as a joystick, keyboard, or remote. This can be facilitated using immersive HMD or a cave augmented virtual environment (CAVE) (Sutherland et al., 2019). A CAVE is a room-sized cube in which projectors or conventional screens are used in conjunction with surround sound to create the immersive VR experience. Recently, limb tracking technology such as the infrared Leap Motion Controller (LMC) has been combined with VR HMD to allow users to see and use a digital representation of their hands for interaction in VR (Backus et al., 2018).

2.6 Telepresence

Finally, telepresence or telemonitoring refers to video conferencing (see Figure 2.4(e)). With telepresence, it is possible to combine a remote experienced physician with a live feed of an operating room containing a display, a video camera on a tripod, and the operating surgeon wearing a headset to guide the attending surgeons though a new surgical technique (Miller et al., 2012).

2.7 RV continuum reference guide

With the taxonomy clearly defined, Figure 2.4 illustrates the taxonomy of the RV continuum according to transportation and artificiality. Transportation in this scenario refers to the extent to which user(s) or object(s) leave behind their local space and enter a remote space (Benford et al., 1998). The figure illustrates the aforementioned display technologies in the RV continuum. The figure has been used as a reference guide to identify computer-mediated reality systems being utilized to solve the needs of clinicians in the IGS process flow depicted in Figure 2.1.

2.8 Image-guided surgery

With the exponential advance in computer technology and the increase of information due to state-of-the-art image processing techniques within hospitals, computer-assisted interventions have become an integral part of any clinician's routine (Mezger et al., 2013). The requirement for computer-assisted interventions was born from the desire to perform safer and less invasive procedures on patients. Image-guided interventions (IGI) are medical procedures that are computer-aided, making use of multi-image modalities to help the physician visualize and target the surgical site. Image-guided surgery (IGS) is the term used for computer-aided interventions that make use of IGI and tracking technology to realize a minimally invasive operation (Hugues et al., 2011). Multimodal images of the patient captured during pre-operative planning, intra-operative guidance, and post-operative review are the central components of IGI and IGS (Alam et al., 2018).

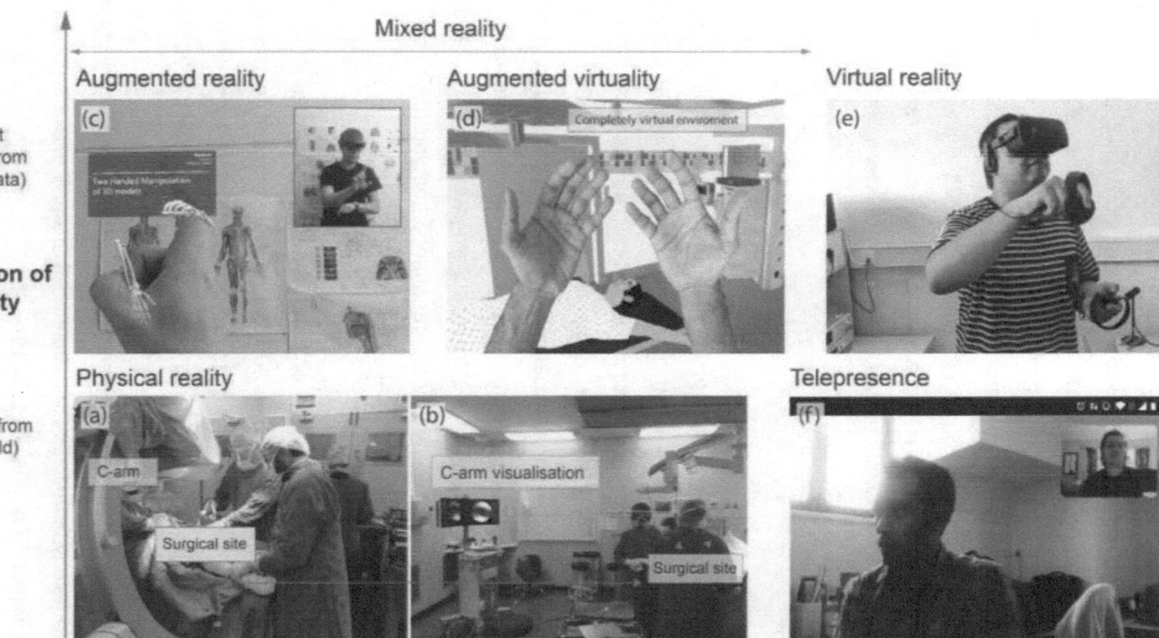

Figure 2.4: Reference guide of the RV continuum with AR, AV, VR and Tele-presence. (a) Groote Schuur operating room with (b) IGS via C-arm visualisation. (c) Author experiencing AR via an AR HMD. (d) A theoretical depiction of AV, a user's hand would have to be visualized realistically in the virtual world whilst wearing a VR HMD configured with an external camera. (d) A medical student wearing a VR HMD to study spatial anatomy. (e) Author and colleague conversing via a telepresence mobile platform.

Figure 2.1. presented earlier shows the cycle of care for any IGS procedure as outlined by Beaulieu et al. (2008). Just like Google maps uses global positioning systems (GPS) to provide visual instruction to a driver by displaying the location of the car on a map, IGS guides the surgeon with real-time feedback about the executed surgical actions through a virtual scene on a display device (Zheng & Nolte, 2015). The physician employs navigational and tracking technology in conjunction with pre-operative or intra-operative images to guide the procedure. Following the patient's and the clinician's user journey through the IGS process flow facilitated the identification of user needs. The following sections discuss each step in the IGS process flow with the identified needs, as well as the computer-mediated reality systems that aim to solve the needs.

2.8.1 Image capture

Pre-operative multimodal images of a region of interest (ROI) allow clinicians to diagnose and plan treatment of various medical problems. Two-dimensional X-ray, ultrasonography (medical ultrasound) and fluoroscopic X-ray as well as three-dimensional (3D) volume modalities such as computed tomography (CT) and magnetic resonance imaging (MRI), are anatomical imaging techniques used for pre-operative imaging. Functional imaging modalities include positron emission tomography (PET), optical imaging, electroencephalogram (EEG) and magnetoencephalogram (MEG), functional magnetic resonance imaging (fMRI) and single-photon emission computed tomography (SPECT).

Depending on the modality, image capture can produce hundreds of images of the patient. For example, a chest CT may have over 500 axial plane images. Any patient movement during image capture can lead to motion artefacts, sometimes necessitating repeat scans (Carlsson et al., 2013). This motivated Liszio et al. (2017) to implement a VR application to prepare patients for scanning procedures, noting a reduction in anxiety and stress which reduced patient movement. Augmented reality systems may also allow radiology technicians to patient positions and relevant patient information for the scans in their FOV (Deebika, 2015).

2.8.2 Visualisation

A variety of visualisation methods have been developed to generate and display 2D images and 3D volumes. For 2D, multiplanar sectioning allows for a slice-by-slice viewing in the axial, sagittal and coronal imaging planes. Whereas for 3D, surface rendering and volume rendering are still the most commonly used methods (Douglas et al., 2018). Without 3D rendering using computer technology, the radiologist must go through each 2D slice and mentally construct a 3D volume. The radiologist's ability to effectively bridge the gap between 2D and 3D is critical to communicating the abnormalities of in the region of interest (ROI) to the clinicians (Douglas et al., 2017). Depending on the intricacy of the anatomy, the interpretation of the scans can be highly challenging, time-consuming, and a point of failure in the IGS process (Cosentino et.al., 2014).

Using AR to view images for diagnostic radiology is currently not Food and Drug Administration (FDA) approved, however, AR stereoscopic displays are supplementing conventional displays and work stations with holographic views (Mandalika et al., 2018) Douglas et al. (2017) reported that radiologists, using a 3D AR HMD system to view a breast CT with a spiculated mass, noted that the shape, margins, and spiculations were better visualized with the AR HMD system than with a conventional 2D display. Clinical scientists are also making use of computational modelling and VR to understand pathologies by virtually immersing themselves in the patient's anatomy (Brouillette et al., 2012). Mandalika et al. (2018) made use of the zSpace display (Figure 2.2) to improve the 3D manipulation required in some diagnostic tasks.

2.8.3 Pre-operative surgical planning

Image-guided interventions use multiple modalities. As such, image registration is required to unite the corresponding positions of multiple patient-specific visualisations. The image registration process assigns correspondences between points on the target images. The entire process can be divided into the following steps: image pre-processing, feature selection and correspondence, determination of transform function, and re-sampling (El-Gamal et al., 2016). During pre-processing the image quality is improved through the correction of scale differences, elimination of motion blur and denoising of images (especially in regions with low contrast objects). Features of an image are the unique characteristics of the image, i.e. the points, corners, lines, curves, templates or regions. Points (landmarks) are the most useful features to determine correspondence and by comparing the coordinates of the matching points a transformation function can be developed to match the geometry of the target images (Alam et al., 2018).

Pre-operative surgical planning includes studying of the visualised image modalities by the clinicians for ascertaining the best procedure to correct the abnormality or injury. Computer-aided surgical simulations have been developed to create models of patient skeletons, dentitions, and soft tissues (Liu et al., 2016). However, 2D displays are noted as the standard means of interacting with the 3D computer models; displays are an integral part of any digital medical imaging system, and previous research has shown that AR/VR HMD 3D user interfaces are more intuitive for navigating volumetric data and enable clinicians to understand spatial relations faster than when interacting with 2D displays (Eck et al., 2016). The idea of using computer-mediated reality techniques for surgical planning is not new; Reitinger et al. (2006) noted that, in neurosurgery, physicians were using AR environments to enhance their interaction and planar perception during the planning process. Augmented reality is frequently used for determining preferred incisions and cutting planes, displaying vital organ information in the surrounding areas, and determining the optimal placement of surgical instruments (Vávra et al., 2017). NOVARAD's Opensight AR system recently became the first medical AR system to receive premarket 510(k) FDA approval (U.S. Food and Drug Administration, 2018). The Opensight system makes use of the Microsoft HoloLens and proprietary software to overlay 2D, 3D, and even four-dimensional (4D) images of the patient's anatomy directly onto the patient's body to aid surgical planning. Currently, these systems only display static images limiting the functional understanding of anatomy such as joints.

2.8.4 Registration for intra-surgical guidance

Registration during IGI or IGS is the alignment of the multiple-image modalities on the 2D displays to the real-world surgical site frame of reference. Intra-operatively, the goal of registration for IGS is to integrate the multimodal images of the patient and the tracked instruments into a common coordinate system. A wide variety of approaches for registration have been developed following numerous methodologies (Zheng et al., 2007). The accuracy and spatial fidelity of the registration are crucial and generally accepted as one of the determining factors of the IGS outcome. The registration between the pre-operative images, the real-world frame of reference and the tracked surgical tools may be prone to inaccuracies due to patient movement, deformation of tissue, or shifting of tracking equipment. Re-registering an inaccurate registration is a lengthy interruption to the surgical procedure and increases the surgical time (Beaulieu et al., 2008).

Registration is an essential component for all computer-mediated reality navigation systems. To register the virtual object or data to the surgical site a variety of registration techniques has been implemented (Chen et al., 2015). The main advantage of using an AR medical system during registration is that the holographic 3D image can be superimposed on the surgical site to improve the calibration process (Hansen et al., 2017). Using AR, the pre-operative image modalities can be manually aligned to anatomical landmarks and skin outlines of the surgical site during user calibration. As an example, Pratt et al. (2018) reported on the superposition of virtual anatomical structures including blood vessels, nerves and bones, onto a patient's limb via the AR optical see-through HMD.

2.8.5 Intra-operative surgical guidance

During minimally invasive surgeries the feedback of the instrument location is particularly useful when the surgeon cannot see the tip of the instrument (Beaulieu et al., 2008). During intra-operative surgical guidance, the surgeon needs to look away from the surgical site to the multimodal imaging data on several displays. The displayed information needs to be combined in context to the surgical site on the patient. This adds mental effort for the surgeon in an already high cognitive load surgery (Sielhorst et al., 2008). Research abounds on how to solve the clinical difficulty of multiple display integration. Solutions include displays mounted on the surgical instruments being used (Herrlich et al., 2017); auditory support for guidance (Hansen et al., 2013) and enhancement of visual displays using AR in surgery (Sielhorst et al., 2008).

Making use of an AR system, surgical tools and digital data sets can be combined into an immersive experience during surgery. Furthermore, the computer-generated images can be superimposed as holograms or mapped overlays onto the surgical site. Multiple studies have validated the use of AR to guide surgeons during minimally invasive surgery (Khor et al., 2016). Currently, the use of AR for surgical guidance has been reported in neurosurgery (Meola et al., 2017), plastic surgery (Kim et al., 2017), orthopaedic surgery (Andress et al., 2018), robotic surgery (Pessaux et al., 2014) and trauma reconstructions (Kim et al., 2017).

As an example, a commercially available IGS system created by SCOPIS medical overlays process guiding visuals onto the live view from the endoscope via the hybrid navigation station's 2D display during endoscopic sinus surgery (Citardi et al., 2016). Gibby et al. (2018) combined NOVARAD's Opensight AR application with an untethered HMD to visualise the pre-operative planned position of pedicle screws. Their AR HMD system guided the placement of pedicle screw through superimposing CT images combined with virtual trajectory guides onto a replica of vertebrae housed in opaque silicone. Their results demonstrated that although there are still several limitations to overcome, the use of an AR HMD had great potential in minimally invasive image-guided interventions.

2.8.6 Post-operative follow-up and rehabilitation

Multi-modal images are used to determine the success of the surgery or treatment during a post-operative follow-up. Postoperative follow-ups are patient-centric, the aim being the verification of a successful surgical outcome, which in turn requires patient care and rehabilitation (Beaulieu et al., 2008). Augmented reality and VR have been used to support remote patient-centred care through games that motivate and guide the patient's rehabilitation exercises (Atrsaei et al. , 2016). Using AR, the patient can see their hands and feet to advance proprioception development with regard to their real environment whilst interacting with the virtual application. Virtual reality has been harnessed to help treat phantom limb pain (Carrino et al., 2014). Several studies demonstrated that by using a VR system, pain experienced by patients during occupational therapy and treatment trials can be mitigated (Pourmand et al., 2018).

Virtual reality is also being utilized to help patients with phobias and mental conditions such as anxiety; the treatment protocol is referred to as virtual reality exposure therapy (Opriş et al., 2012).

2.9 Other use cases of computer-mediated reality systems

Surgery and procedural training, the study of human biomechanics (Voinea et al., 2016) and telemedicine (an economical and effective solution to address the problem of training health care providers in remote locations) are notable fields of development for computer-mediated reality. Augmented reality systems can be developed to provide a platform for enabling the recording of surgeries as well as the creation of training simulations to deliver surgical expertise and impart surgical skills (Kim et al., 2017). Computer-mediated reality systems have also been used to show patients possible outcomes from plastic surgery with virtual aesthetics visualisations (Khor et al., 2016).

With combining AR and telemedicine, the FOV of an attending surgeon can be broadcast to a second surgeon, located remotely, empowered with a virtual interactive presence and augmented reality (VIPAR) system. The VIPAR system allows the remote surgeon to place their hands in the recorded footage which is streamed back to the attending surgeon. The surgeon can interact with this hybrid AR image using an AR HMD, which combines the real environment view with a holographic representation of a colleague's hands in real-time (Shenai et al., 2011). Gross anatomy education (Kugelmann et al., 2018) is also a notable field. Functional understanding is being established by creating a biomechanical model or "rig" of the patient's movements combined with the computer-generated visualisation using external tracking technology (Blum et al., 2012).

2.10 Summary

The use of computer-mediated reality systems in the medical field is receiving increased research attention (Kersten-Oertel et al., 2016). As discussed, computer-mediated reality systems can potentially improve the user's experience in each step of the IGS workflow, specifically pre-surgical planning, intra-operative guidance, post-surgical assessment and rehabilitation. For the surgical application, AR could aid in reducing the cognitive overload experienced by clinicians due to integrating multi-modal imaging data from several sources while performing the intervention on the patient. By superimposing the virtual image data into the user's field of view, the cognitive load experienced due to switching between monitors and the surgical site identified in conventional surgery can be resolved. The following chapter details the systems required to create an intra-operative surgical guiding AR HMD medical system.

Chapter 3: Augmented reality to enhance the field of view of the clinician

This chapter presents the essential functional, technical and technological requirements to create an AR medical system where the virtual objects (or data) are registered to a specified location in the real environment.

3.1 Intra-operative surgical guidance AR medical system

As described in the preceding chapter, computer-mediated reality technologies have the potential to improve all processes in the IGS workflow. For intra-operative surgical guidance, employing AR technology for FOV enhancement has been suggested as a method to aid in reducing the cognitive overload experienced by clinicians. The cognitive overload can be attributed to the necessity of integrating multi-modal imaging data from several sources while performing the image-guided intervention on the patient. Locally (South Africa), the need for an AR technology for IGS was confirmed through observing surgical orthopaedic procedures performed at Groote Schuur Hospital and University of Cape Town (Figure 3.1).

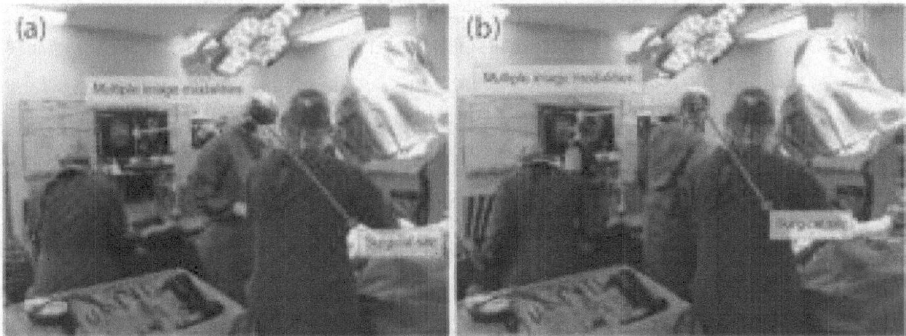

Figure 3.1: Groote Schuur OR with C-arm. As shown by the arrows the attending physician is required to integrate multi-modal imaging data from several sources while performing the intervention on the patient. (a) The surgeon is looking towards the surgical site. (b) The surgeon has turned around to few the multiple-image modalities.

As stated in chapter 2, AR uses an electronic display or projection module to add computer-generated data to the user's FOV. For intra-operative surgical guidance (further referred to as intra-surgical guidance) the user/s is/are the attending clinician(s). The utility of an intra-surgical AR medical system is that the procedural guidance imagery can be displayed as an apparent holographic image on the surgical site as opposed to the common visualization techniques on multiple displays (Navab et al., 2007). Soler et al. (2014) stated that augmenting the FOV of the clinician with patient-specific data to aid in surgical guidance is based on two major processes, namely, the 3D modelling and visualization of the anatomical or pathological structures identified in the region of interest (ROI), and the registration of the visualization onto the real patient. The patient data to be visualized will be referred to as the virtual object.

3.2 Intra-surgical guidance AR medical system requirements

The transformation from one Cartesian coordinate system to another, also called registration, is required to enable intra-surgical guidance with image modalities (Meulstee et al., 2019). As stated in chapter 2, the goal of registration for IGS is to integrate unimodal or multimodal images of the patient and the tracked instruments into a common coordinate system.

For an intra-surgical guidance AR medical system, the patient-specific data must be registered accurately; failing this the clinician could be misled and cause serious harm. As such, in theory, the accuracy of the registration for intra-surgical guidance should be sub-millimetre, however, most current AR medical system research projects report accuracy within millimetres (Chen et al., 2017). Although the second and third set of requirements from Table 2.1 (see chapter 2 section 7) describes the alignment of a virtual and real-world object, further expansion of the functional and technical requirements are required to highlight the importance of registering the virtual object (modality visualization) to the pose (location and orientation) of the real-world object (surgical site) for the intra-surgical guidance use case.

It should be noted that the display module and the perceived location of the visualization are limited by the physical constraints of the operating room which include the need for sterile equipment, the freedom of movement of the surgeon, and harsh lighting conditions. As such, the functional and technical requirements may be updated as follows (Table 3.1) for an intra-surgical guidance AR medical system:

Table 3.1: Functional requirements vs. technical requirements required for an AR medical system for intra-surgical guidance.

Nr.	Functional Requirement	Technical requirement
1.	A sterile AR system that runs interactively, allows freedom of movement, and user (clinician) interactions in real-time.	The 3D visualization needs to the viewable from several positions, merged with the real-time view of the user (clinician), and respond to the user's inputs to not interfere with the sterility of the AR medical system.
2.	The virtual object (modality visualization) needs to be registered in 3D to the real-world object (surgical site).	A tracking and registration system to resolve the pose (location and orientation) of the real-world object and register the corresponding virtual object onto this location.
3.	The required location (i.e. surgical site) and the virtual content should be combined in an operating room.	A tracking system that can determine the FOV of the user(clinician) and display the superimposed view of the virtual object onto the real-world object with high accuracy in harsh lighting conditions.

3.3 Typical architecture of an AR medical system to solve for intra-surgical guidance

It is a standard software application development practice to refer to an undeveloped system as a black box (Beizer et al., 1995). This is done to identify key processes required of a system between inputs and the outputs. From Table 4.2 we can determine the inputs and output of the intra-surgical guidance AR medical system. For inputs, at least four sources of information can be discerned, namely:

1. The patient data to be visualized.
2. The real-world footage of the user (clinician).
3. The user's (clinician's) FOV pose data.
4. The pose data of the real-world object (i.e. surgical site).

Figure 3.2 illustrates the typical system architecture of an AR medical system to solve for intra-surgical guidance with regard to the specified inputs, the black box and the output. For the output, the desired outcome is the superimposed AR view of the virtual object registered onto the surgical site in 3D. The output is facilitated by combining the computed virtual object with the real-world footage to render the AR visualization via a display to the user (clinician). The black box needs to consist of multiple technological modules and processes working in tandem to process the given system inputs into the required output. This typically includes modules for image capture, tracking modules; image processing, computer vision, and virtual object computing (Daponte et al., 2014).

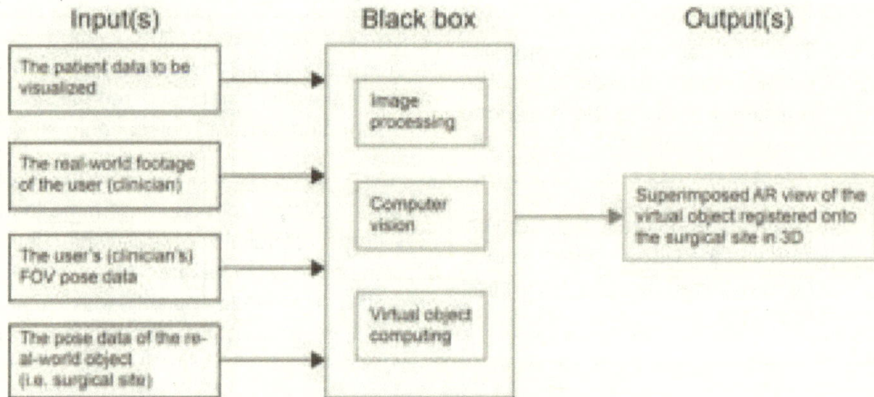

Figure 3.2: The typical architecture of the AR medical system to superimpose a virtual object in situ represented as a Black Box system.

To solve for the required output from the inputs, the black box needs to combine the technological modules and processes to complete the following key processes.

1. Spatially map the real-world scene.
2. Identify the current FOV of the user (clinician).
3. Determine the location of the real-world object in the real-world scene.
4. Determine the scale and pose of the virtual object (virtual object computing).

The combined modules and processes identified all act as supersets for several tasks and technological systems. Their technological requirements and subsets are discussed in the following sections.

3.4. The patient data to be visualized

3.4.1 The source of the visualization

The raw medical images sources can be MRI or CT or ultrasonography in the digital imaging and communication in medicine (DICOM) standard (Kersten-Oertel et al., 2012). It is important that the patient's positioning during the scan procedure matches the intervention procedure position. Adherence will mitigate the effect of anatomical deformation between acquisition time and intervention to minimise registration inaccuracies of the computer-generated graphic (Pratt et al., 2018): If the real data source changes with time, the computer-generated graphics need to be updated accordingly, as is the case during fluoroscopy IGS procedures (Andress et al., 2018).

3.4.2 Creating the virtual object

The standard DICOM patient-based coordinate system assumes a subject is imaged in the supine position. The DICOM coordinate system is in a right-handed orientation basis, with the X-axis going from the right to the left of the patient, the Y-axis from the front of the patient to the back (anterior to posterior) and the Z-axis goes from the feet of the patient to the head of the patient (inferior to superior). This is denoted to as the Left, Posterior, Superior (LPS) 3D basis. Different medical applications use different definitions of this 3D basis. Depending on the use case, the raw DICOM images are transformed from the 2D datasets (left to right and top to bottom) to a voxel-based 3D volume rendering of the required anatomical structures with the medical image processing software. The voxel-based 3D volume file size can be large, which can lead to latency during virtual object processing (Kang et al., 2014). As such, using medical image processing software, the 3D volume rendering is often converted to a polygon-based 3D volume.

3.4.3 The virtual world scene

The polygon-based 3D volume is manipulated with 3D computer graphics software to smooth the mesh and enhance the “realism” of the virtual object. The manipulated 3D volume is then added to a 3D world game engine or scene generator application, where a virtual world coordinate system is created. It is common practice to assign a point of origin of the FOV in the virtual world scene. The FOV is known as the virtual camera in the 3D world game engine application. The virtual object is positioned around the virtual camera point of origin in the virtual world scene coordinate frame. As such there are three transformation matrices that are implemented on the original voxel-based 3D volume coordinate frame: the DICOM to 3D computer graphics software, the 3D computer graphics to the 3D game engine application, and the relation of the virtual object to the virtual camera in the virtual world coordinate system. These transformation matrices contain information about the position, orientation and scale of the 3D volume.

3.5 Manipulation of the remaining inputs to solve the key processes identified

3.5.1 Capturing and processing of the real-world footage

To create an AR visualization, a recording device needs to capture the real environment. Recording devices that have been reported in the literature for capturing the real environment are hand-held cameras, head-mounted cameras and depth-cameras (Daponte et al., 2014). Computer vision makes use of the captured images (video) to determine a required set of variables, during processes such as spatial mapping of the real-world scene, FOV determination, and identifying the location of the real-world object in the real-world scene. As such it could be said that the camera acts as an “electronic eye” (Sherman et al., 2018). The difference between computer vision and image processing are the goals. Image processing manipulates the image or video to change its form or state. Computer vision makes use of the changed state of the image or video in combination with an array of tracking sensor modules to calculate the required set of variables.

To allow for the real-world scene spatial mapping, FOV calculation, image processing, and computer vision, the components typically required are central processing units (CPU), graphics processing units (GPU), an array of tracking sensor modules, and the aforementioned 3D world game engine application. Typically, the 3D world game engine application is used to create a virtual world scene that mimics the real-world scene. As such, the scale of the virtual world scene for an AR application depends on the required user experience.

The aforementioned camera and tracking modules can either be "external" to the display module (outside-in tracking) or combined into a single unit (inside-out tracking). In the case of HMDs and handheld displays (smartphones), the video camera is built-in with the rest of the modules. As such, HMD and smartphones are examples of inside-out tracking systems. The difference between the Cartesian coordinate systems of the video-camera module, the tracking modules, and the display module are negligible (Daponte et al., 2014). This allows the Cartesian coordinate systems of the three modules to be consolidated into one coordinate system - the FOV of the user (clinician).

3.5.2 Spatial mapping of the real-world scene

There are two critical processes that need to run simultaneously upon launching the AR application; the spatial mapping of the real environment and the localization of the FOV point of origin. This is classified as simultaneous localization and mapping (SLAM) (Vassallo et al., 2017).

Spatial mapping describes the process of combining the tracking module data about the FOV and the data from the real-time footage to recreate a virtual mesh of the environment. Spatial mapping is a form of computer vision that specifically determines the distance, depth, and orientation of the objects seen in the real-world scene. These captured variables are used to calculate the pose of the user's FOV and the pose of the real-world object in regard to the real-world scene's Cartesian coordinate system.

3.5.3 Determining the FOV

The tracking sensor modules are used in combination with the real-world footage to determine the FOV of the clinician. Tracking the FOV of the clinician is accomplished by combining inertial measurement unit (IMU) sensors, computer vision algorithms, infrared sensors, ultrasonic sensors or combinations of the above (Daponte et al., 2014). Irrespective of the technology, determining the FOV comprises two phases: (1) a registration phase which determines the pose of the user (clinician) with regard to the real environment; (2) a tracking phase which updates the pose of the user (clinician) relative to the previously known pose. The term tracking refers to the combined application of both phases. The captured information is represented as the six-degree-of-freedom (6-DOF) values (Sherman et al., 2018), which are represented in Table 3.2 and illustrated in Figure 3.3 around a user (clinician) wearing an HMD below.

Table 3.2: The 6-DOF values

Position or location	**The orientation angles**
X (forward and back)	Pitch
Y (up and down)	Roll
Z (left and right) coordinates.	Yaw

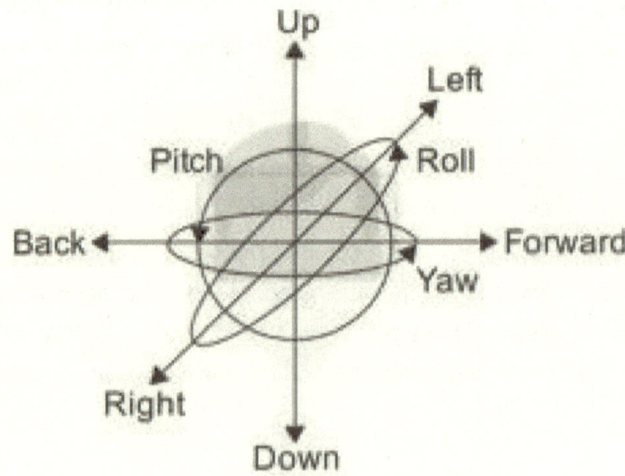

Figure 3.3: Depiction of the 6-DOF values around an HMD.

3.5.4 Determining the pose of the real-world object

User calibration (Pratt et al., 2018) and optical tracking systems have been reported as solutions for registration in combination with AR medical systems (Chen et al., 2015). Optical tracking systems include fiducial marker tracking systems (Müller et al., 2013) and markerless tracking systems (Wang et al. , 2019).

3.5.4.1 User calibration for registration

User calibration is not an automated registration process. The virtual object is rendered to the clinician according to its location specified in the virtual world scene. The clinician has to manipulate the scale and orientation of the virtual object to match the location and landmark features of the real-world object being augmented in the real-world scene (Katić et al., 2015).

3.5.4.2 Fiducial marker tracking systems

In IGS, an optical tracking system is often used to integrate the multimodal images of the patient and the tracked instruments into a common coordinate system. The optical tracking system combines infrared (IR) light-emitting diodes (LED) with two monochromatic cameras at a fixed distance to each other (Azimi et al., 2017). Active markers have IR light-emitting diodes built-in, whereas passive markers need to be coated with an infrared light retroreflecting material. The optical tracking sensor determines the pose of the real-world object by measuring the amount of light that is transmitted by or reflected from the fiducial markers placed on the tracked object (Preim et al., 2013).

A subset of fiducial marker-based tracking systems makes use of computer vision to identify predefined features of template markers from the recorded footage using image processing algorithms. In other words, the camera (the optical system) capturing the real-world footage acts as an "electronic eye". Template markers are normally a set of patterns that are easily distinguishable (Figure 3.4). The pose of the virtual object is specified in the virtual scene in relation to the fiducial marker (active or passive) in the 3D world game engine application (Frantz et al., 2018). The virtual object is then placed according to the specified pose in the real-world scene when the marker is identified in the real-world footage.

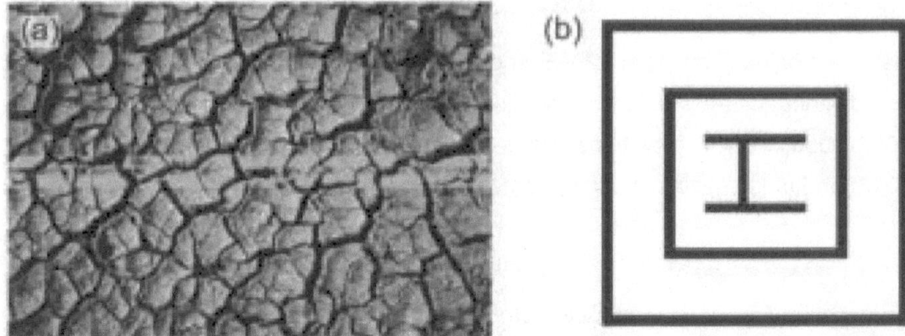

Figure 3.4: Examples of target images for marker vision-based tracking. (a) The (a) The Vuforia tarmac target image (Frantz et al., 2018). *(b) A template marker with clear patterns created by the author.*

3.5.4.3 Markerless tracking systems

A more complex version of optical tracking is markerless or feature-based tracking. Here the marker is inferred or deduced with computer vision (Szeliski, 2011). Depending on the scale of the real-world scene and accuracy required, a monocular or stereo (Schoob et al., 2017) based camera system is required. Computer vision techniques are used to determine the location of the real-world object according to what the camera "sees" (Sherman et al., 2018). As an example, by combining image processing with 3D scanning and matching algorithms (Wang et al., 2019) a computer vision technique is established. Another example of a computer vision technique is a convolutional neural network that has been developed and trained to recognise the key features of the real-world object in the video footage (Zhang et al., 2019).

3.5.5 Virtual object computing

By combining the first three process variables, spatial mapping, FOV, and information of the real-world object, the pose and scale of the virtual object required in the real scene can be computed (virtual object computing). The FOV and pose data of the real-world object are transferred to the virtual world scene Cartesian coordinate system to determine the required virtual object. To create the AR visualization, the computed virtual object needs to be combined with the real-world footage to be rendered via a form of a display to the user (clinician). As mentioned, both image processing and computer vision techniques are required to determine the pose of the real-world object from the real-world footage and merge the real-world footage with the virtual object.

3.6 The output - computed computer graphics rendered through a display

In terms of creating the final AR visualization, the goal of image processing is to combine the computed virtual object with the recorded footage to be rendered to the clinician via the display module. The recorded footage is made transparent and combined with the virtual object to be rendered into the user's FOV using the video display module or projector as an apparent holographic AR 3D volume. This means that the clinician can see the 3D virtual objects as an apparent opaque hologram, interact with the virtual object, and view it from every angle.

Important requirements for medical AR visualizations are high-resolution displays and rendering frame rates higher than what the eye can see. For realistic rendering, a minimum frame rate of 30 frames per second (fps) is required (Chen et al., 2017). High latency decreases the performance of the system and can influence the frame rate of the AR view (Dey et al., 2018). If the rendering frame rate drops below the 30fps the refreshing and rendering of the virtual object will be seen. This would distract the user (clinician) from the usefulness of the AR medical system. Recent advances in smartphone-powered video see-through HMD, as described in chapter 2 section 3.6, have reached the specified requirements. However, video see-through HMDs have been reported to induce inaccurate depth perception and nausea (Sielhorst et al., 2008). As such, optical see-through HMD or Spatial AR displays are the recommended platforms for intra-surgical guidance (Yoon et al., 2018).

3.7 Assessing an AR medical system

The literature shows that the analysis of current AR medical systems focuses on the errors, accuracy, visual perception, and the user's experience (Dey et al., 2018). The performance of the AR medical system can be assessed according to the alignment of the AR visualization to the required real environment (Chen et al., 2015), the depth of perception of the AR visualization (Diaz et al., 2017), or the speed of tracking and rendering (Daponte et al., 2014). The visual perception of the AR visualization focuses on the quality of the visualization to enable depth perception (Gabbard et al. , 2010). User experience assessment of an AR medical system includes accessing the ability of the AR visualization to add insight (level of information enhancement) or the intuitiveness of the graphical UI.

3.8 Summary

Figure 3.5 shows the required architecture of an AR medical system to enhance the FOV of a clinician wearing an HMD with the virtual object registered about the patient. For the AR medical system to run seamlessly, real environment capturing, tracking, and registration and rendering of the computer-generated data via the display need to run simultaneously. The components and systems running in unison are highlighted by the multi-directional arrows in Figure 3.5. With all the specifications, requirements, and assessment criteria of an AR medical system specified, the developed proof of concept AR HMD systems can be discussed in the following chapter.

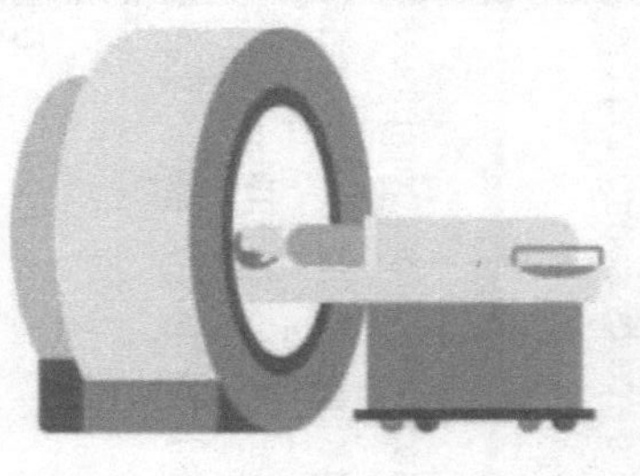

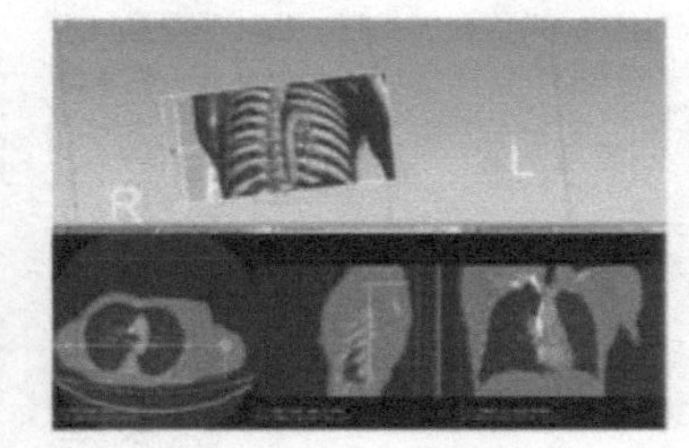

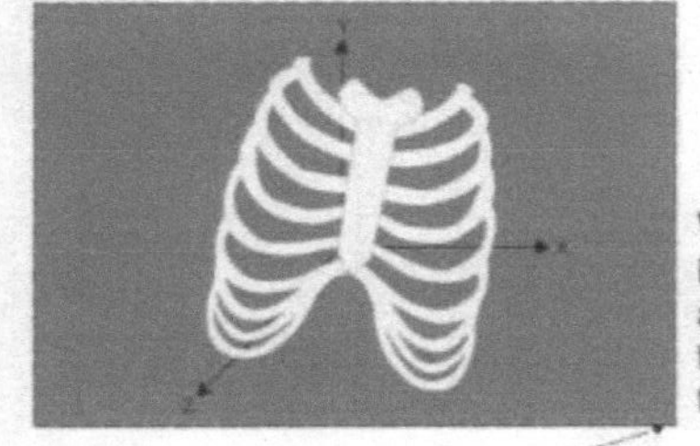

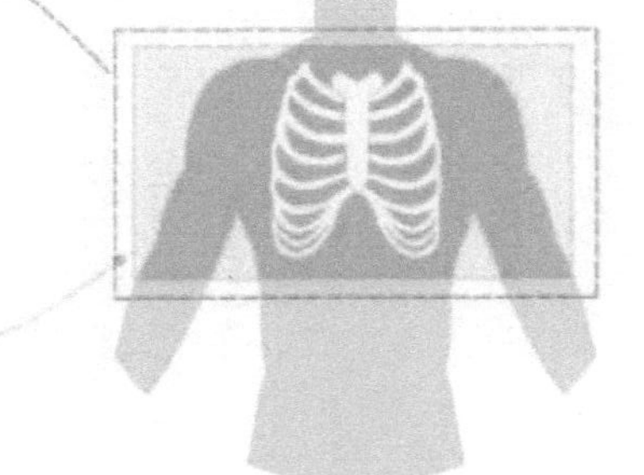

Figure 3.5: The system architecture of an AR HMD medical system to visualize patient-specific data in the FOV of the surgeon. For the AR HMD medical system to run seamlessly, the image capturing, tracking, localization and displaying of the AR view need to run in unison.

Chapter 4: Overview of the augmented reality medical system

This project aimed to develop an AR HMD medical system to aid intra-surgical guidance. For such a system, aligning the virtual object to the surgical site is one of the key requirements. Head-mounted displays are the recommended platforms for intra-surgical guidance (Yoon et al., 2018). Current off-the-shelf untethered optical see-through AR devices such as the Microsoft HoloLens and Magic Leap (www.magicleap.com) are constantly improving to address the pre-requisites for AR visual enhancement as discussed in chapter 3 (Kolodzey et al., 2017).

Both these devices use see-through mirror optical lenses to reflect the computer-generated images, thereby combining the real and virtual world views. Currently, HoloLens is considered to be one of the most suitable AR HMD devices for surgical practice (Qian et al., 2017). This chapter describes the proof-of-concept AR HMD systems developed with the HoloLens.

4.1 The Microsoft HoloLens

The HoloLens is a complete AR HMD system that has an array of sensors with adequate computing power to create AR experiences. The user can operate the device using voice or hand gestures. The HoloLens can display apparent holograms with a frame rate of up to 60 Hz (60 FPS). The user's FOV is augmented with the apparent holographic 3D visuals by rendering high-quality computed graphics into the optical see-through waveguide display lenses. The diffractive waveguide in the display lenses guides the light waves into the optical path of the user's eye by controlling the internal reflection of the light between entry and exit (Qian et al., 2017).

Computational processing is handled by the Cherry Trail-based Intel Atom combined CPU/GPU 32-bit processor and a coprocessor, Microsoft's internally developed Holographic Processing Unit (HPU). The HPU handles the integration of environmental data and user input (gaze, gesture and voice). Propriety algorithms combine the spatial and tracking information from the inertial measurement unit (IMU) (which includes an accelerometer, gyroscope, and a magnetometer), the four "environment understanding" cameras, and one depth camera (time-of-flight depth sensors) to map the direct environment and determine the pose of the HMD, i.e. simultaneous localization and mapping (El-Hariri et al., 2018). The key technical specifications of the HoloLens (Generation one) to capture the real environment footage, the pose of the HMD, and render the holographic visuals are summarized in Table 4.1.

Table 4.1: Microsoft HoloLens system specification.

Classification	**Technical specification**
Design specifications	120 degrees FOV. 2-3 hours battery (active use). Weight is 580g.
Hardware specifications	Intel 32-bit architecture with TPM 2.0 support. Memory: 2 GB RAM 64 GB flash. Custom-built Microsoft Holographic Processing Unit (HPU)
Communication	Bluetooth 4.1LE Wi-Fi 802.11ac Micro USB 2.0
Sensors	2 mega-pixel camera / high definition (HD) video camera. 1 x depth camera. 1 x ambient light sensor. 1 x IMU.
The optical see-through display specifications (Figure 4.8)	2 x see-through holographic lenses (waveguides). 2 x HD 16:9 light engines. Automatic pupillary distance calibration. Holographic Resolution: 2.3 million total light points. Holographic Density: >2.5k radiant (light points per radian).

4.2 The hand as a clinical example for IGS

With the HoloLens selected as the AR platform to explore the development of an AR HMD medical system, an IGS procedure needed to be selected to assess the registration accuracy of the virtual object (patient data) to its corresponding real-world object (surgical site). Mutilating hand injuries present significant challenges for the hand surgeon and the patient. Damage to the associated soft tissue and combination of fractures make each hand injury unique. The pre-surgical visualization and intra-surgical guidance requirements for hand surgeries match the needs identified in chapter 2 and so can possibly be solved using an AR HMD medical system. Combined with the manageable size, easily distinguishable landmarks, and the complexity of the biomechanical movement of the hand, the hand makes for a useful clinical example of IGS. The following sections detail the anatomy of the hand; the biomechanical complexity of the hand; and clinical procedures related to the hand which would benefit from an AR HMD medical system.

4.2.1 Anatomy of the wrist and hand

The hand is a multi-digit appendage located at the end of the forearm that forms part of the upper limb appendicular skeleton of the human musculoskeletal system. The bones of the upper limb from proximal to distal are specified as the scapula, clavicle, humerus, radius, ulna, wrist and hand (Figure 4.1). The functions of the hand require the interaction of muscles, tendons, bones, joints and nerves (Lee et al., 2015). The wrist comprises of two rows of small carpals bones of different shape; eight bones in total. The carpal bones in the proximal row articulate with the radius to form the wrist joint. The distal end of the ulna does not directly articulate with any of the carpal bones.

The wrist is also referred to as the base of the hand (Figure 4.2). The carpal bones form a u-shaped grouping with the flexor retinaculum spanning this u-shaped area to maintain the grouping of the carpal bones and form the carpal tunnel (Betts et al., 2013). The tendons that allow flexing of the hand, as well as the median nerve, pass through this area. The flexor retinaculum is attached laterally to the scaphoid bone that gives support to the thumb (pollex). The scaphoid bone allows for the opposition and reposition of the hand.

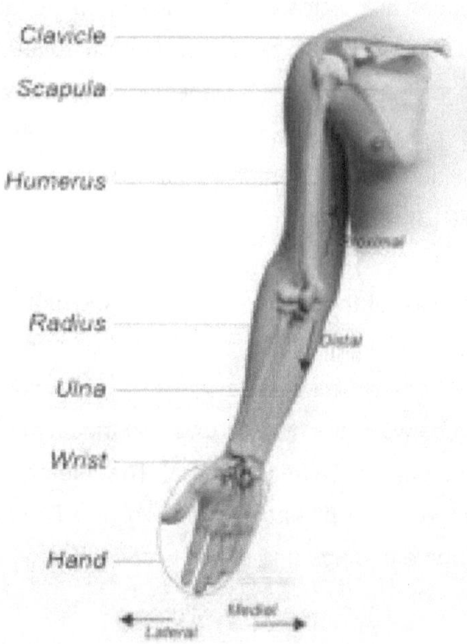

Figure 4.1: Anterior view of the upper limb, bones, and anatomical positions. The image is a rendering of the Atomedge model.

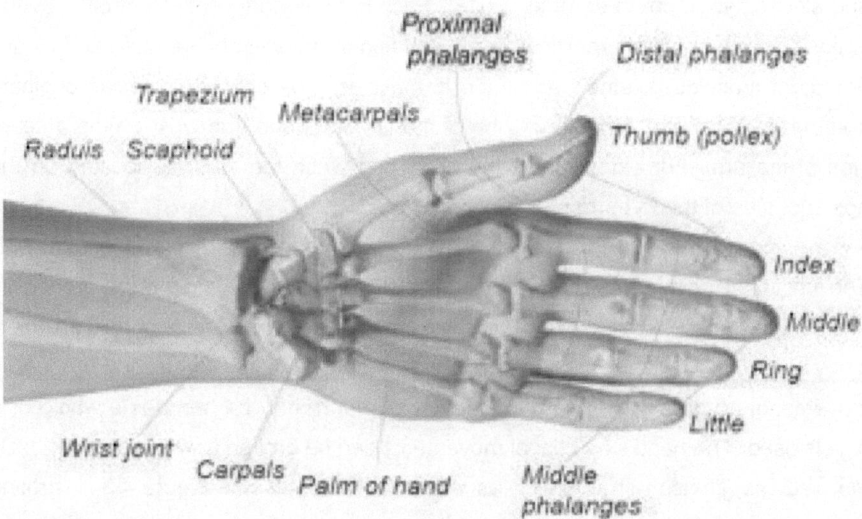

Figure 4.2: Anterior view of arm, wrist and hand detailing key anatomical features. The image is a rendering of the Atomedge model.

The distal row of carpal bones articulates with the base of the metacarpals to form the carpometacarpal joints. The palm of the hand consist of five metacarpal bones. The first metacarpal bone is located between the trapezium and proximal phalanx of the thumb and is separated from the other metacarpal bones by intrinsic muscle tissue and facia. This spacing allows independent freedom of movement of the thumb from the fingers (Betts et al., 2013).

The thumb and fingers consist of the fourteen phalanx bones. The thumb (pollex) is digit number one and consists of two phalanges. Digit two (index finger) to digit five (little finger) all have three phalanges each, namely the proximal, middle and distal phalanx bones. The joints between the metacarpals and the proximal phalanx of each digit are referred to as metacarpophalangeal joints. The interphalangeal joint is the articulation point between adjacent phalanges of the digits. The fingers of the hand contain a dense area of nerve endings and are the richest source of tactile feedback (Lachapelle, 2014).

4.2.2 The biomechanical motion of the hand

Biomechanical study of the human hand includes anthropometry, kinematics, kinetics, and electromyography (Lee et al., 2013). Each hand is dominantly controlled by the opposing brain hemisphere. Wrist, hand, and finger movements are facilitated by two groups of muscles, extrinsic and intrinsic muscles. The extrinsic muscles originate from the forearm and allow for flexion of the fingers, hand and wrist on the anterior side of the arm. For extension of the hand and wrist, the muscles located on the posterior side of the forearm need to be activated.

The functional movements of the hand can be divided into two main groups, prehensile and non-prehensile. Prehensile movements are gestures which seize or hold an object partly or wholly within the compartment of the hand. During non-prehensile movements no grasping or seizing is involved, but rather the hand as a whole or a digit is used. The hand's functional movements can be broken down into seven basic manoeuvres (Duncan et al., 2013) as shown in Table 4.2 with Figure 4.3 illustrating the movement of the hand and the joints.

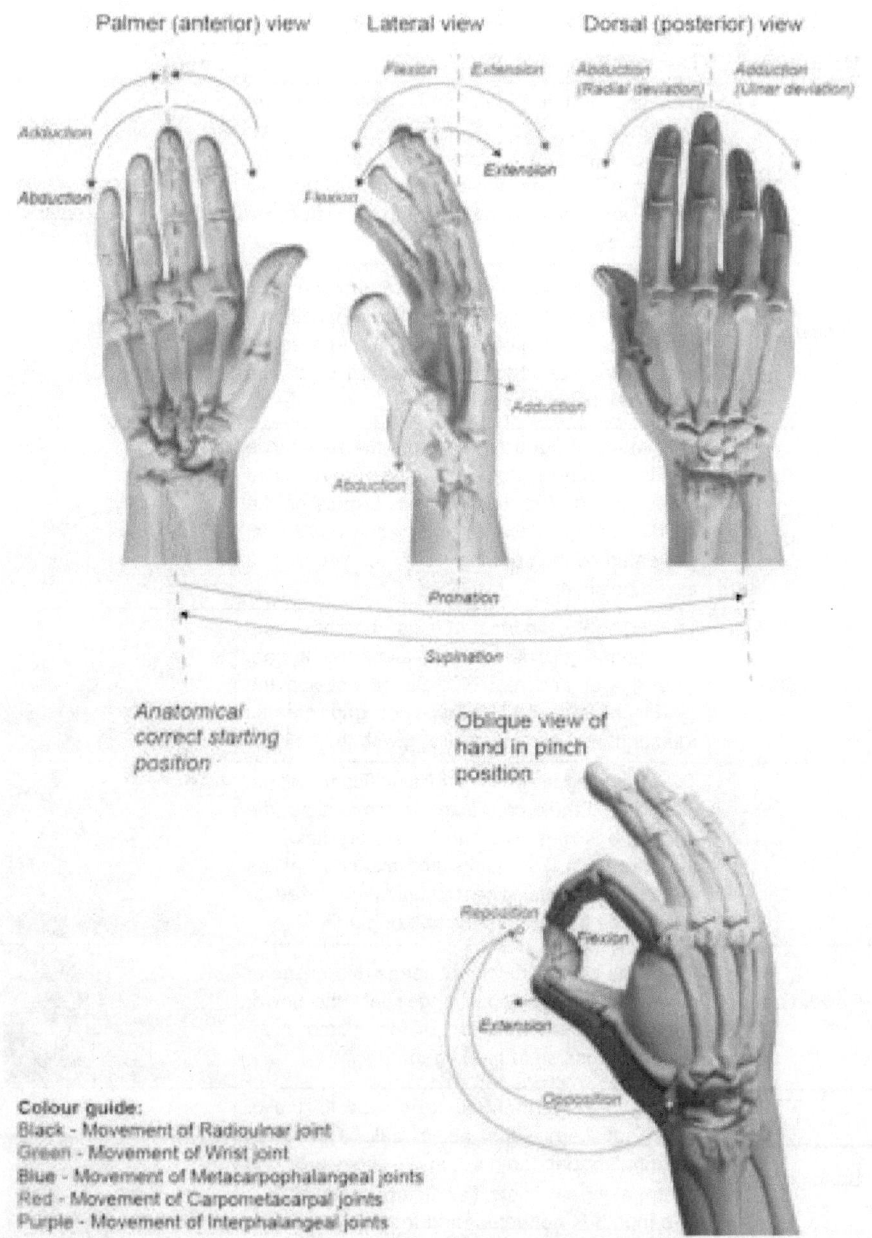

Figure 4.3: Multiple views of the right hand to illustrate the movements of the respective joints found in the wrist and hand. The image is a rendering of the Atomedge model.

Table 4.2: The seven basic hand functions (Duncan et al., 2013).

Manoeuvre	Description	Image
Precision pinch	The tips of the thumb and index finger are brought together so that a small item such as a card or pen can be picked up. Bringing the thumb and index finger together is termed opposition and moving the thumb away from the index finger is reposition.	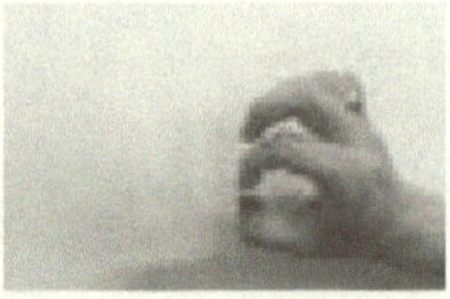
Oppositional pinch	The pulp of the index finger and thumb are used to hold the pre-defined item with an oppositional pinch. The holding of the item is made possible through increased forces generated by thumb and index finger opposition.	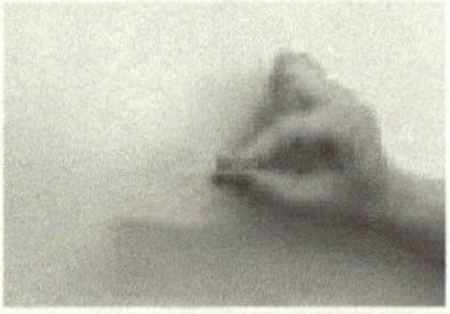
Key pinch	The thumb is adducted towards the radial side of the index finger during key pinch manoeuvring. The thumb exerts a force on the middle phalanx of the index finger. A stable post is created by the keeping rest of the fingers in a flexed position.	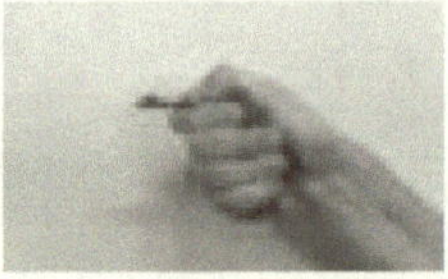
Chuck grip	To hold light cylindrical objects, the chuck grip (directional grip) is used to allow the thumb, index finger and rest of digits to envelop the cylindrical object. This type of grip creates rotational and axial force along with the object.	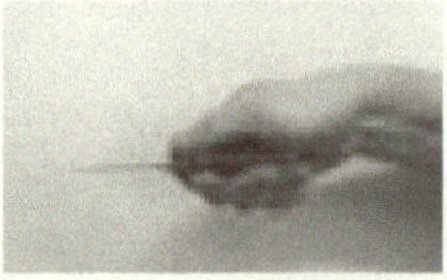
Hook grip	To lift cylindrical objects of significant weight, such as a handle connected to a briefcase, the hook grip is required. The fingers are flexed at the interphalangeal joints and extended at the metacarpal joints. The thumb is not used to exert force but acts as a stabilizing unit.	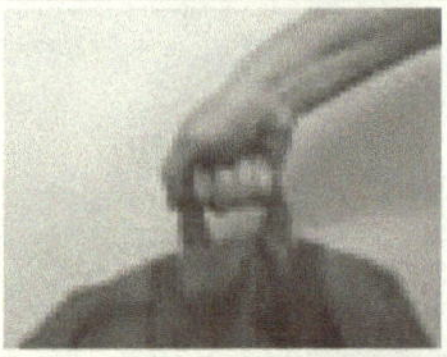
Power Grasp	When the cylindrical object needs to be used or moved, the hook grip changes into the power grasp to allow for flexion of the thumb in an opposed position to the fingers.	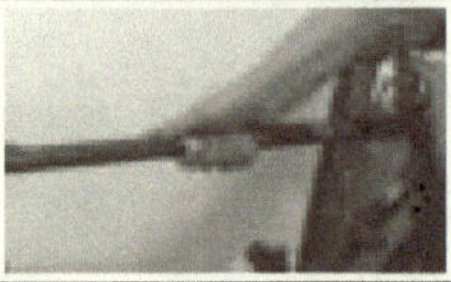
Span grasp	The span grasp manoeuvre is used to grip or catch an item such as a ball. The distal interphalangeal joints and the proximal interphalangeal joints flex to an angle of 30°. The thumb is abducted, and force is generated by the thumb and fingers on the object.	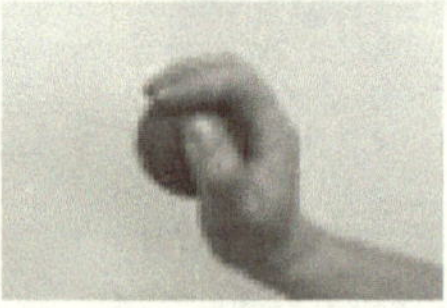

4.2.3 Injuries and treatment of hand trauma

A thorough understanding of the biomechanical impact of a hand injury is required for the making of decisions during the treatment of hand trauma (Baltzer et al., 2016). When the severity of a hand injury results in surgery, the hand's ability to manipulate the positions listed in Table 4.2 as well as the ability to exert the correct biomechanical force to allow for functional movements determines the success of the procedure. Mutilating hand injuries vary in magnitude and severity (Tosti et al., 2018).

Most hand injuries occur on the bones of the hand and treatment guidelines have been developed for the most common fractures types. Phalangeal and metacarpal fractures are among the most common skeletal injuries (Green et al., 2016). Mutilating hand injuries present significant challenges for the hand surgeon and the patient. The severe damage to the associated soft tissue and combination of fractures makes each hand injury unique. The surgeon often needs to make decisions during surgery directly after initial debridement of the hand as to finger and joint preservation to ensure hand function (Baltzer et al., 2016).

The role of imaging with traumatic hand and finger injuries is to aid the diagnosis of the injury type to allow the emergency physicians and orthopaedic surgeons to plan the correct treatment. Surgical techniques on the hand that use IGS include arthroplasty, avascular necrosis, carpal tunnel syndrome release surgery, minimally invasive finger fracture management as well as trauma treatment of open and closed hand injuries (Bowen et al., 2014).

The imaging modality of choice for these procedures is radiography (X-rays) with a minimal of three angle views; these include posteroanterior, oblique and lateral views (Sheehan et al., 2016). Magnetic resonance imaging, ultrasonographic and CT procedures are also used depending on the severity of bone or soft tissue injury.

4.3 The virtual and real-world objects

With hand and wrist injury treatments to be explored as the example IGS process flow, an equivalent virtual object was required of the lower arm. As such, an anatomically correct 3D arm model developed by Atomedge Solutions was acquired to be used as the virtual object. The propriety anatomical model was created from multiple 3D scans and X-ray images.

4.3.1 The anatomically correct arm model

Atomedge Solutions combined the following software packages to create the anatomically correct hand model 1.) NextEngine Scan Studio for 3D scanning and processing; 2.) Pixologic Zbrush for 3D sculpting and texture painting; 3.) and Autodesk 3DS Max for modelling, rendering and exporting of the computer graphic (Figure 4.4 (a) and (b)).

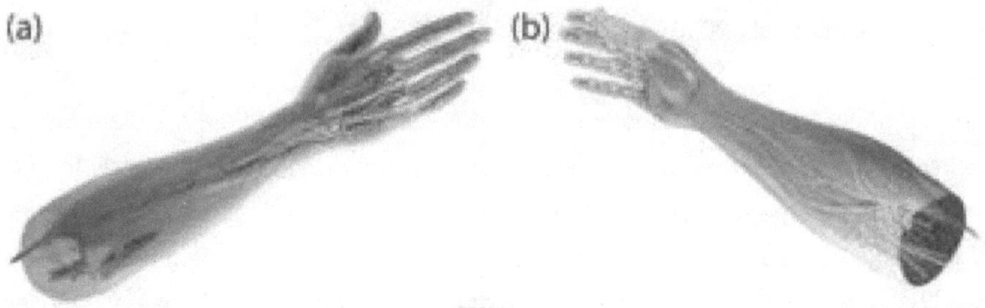

Figure 4.4: Renders of the anatomically correct model developed by Atomedge. (a) Posterior view of Atomedge complex anatomical model. (b) Anterior view Atomedge complex anatomical model.

The anatomical model was simplified to the skin and bone structures using Autodesk Inventor (2018). The file size of the simplified.OBJ 3D volume was 3267 KB. The anatomically correct 3D arm is part of a full-body model created by Atomedge Solutions as part of a previous project, using cadaver images obtained under ethics approval HREC REF 595/2015.

4.3.2 The real-world object

To validate the registration of the aforementioned virtual object to a real-world object, a 3D printed hand of the skin layer was fabricated using a Zortax M200 3D printer (https://zortrax.com/) with black filament (Figure 4.5).

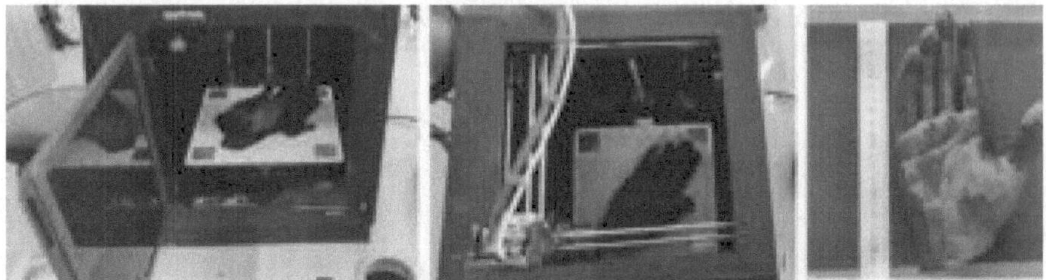

Figure 4.5: The 3D printed hand of the Atomedge anatomically correct hand model.

4.3.3 Exploring virtual object creation from the real data source

To explore the creation of a virtual object form patient-specific data and using it to enhance the FOV of the clinician, a 3D bone geometry of a patient's hand was extracted from a full-body computed tomography angiography scan of a patient acquired at the Groote Schuur Hospital in Cape Town. Ethical clearance to use the image data was obtained from the University of Cape Town's Human Research Ethics Committee HREC REF 458/2018. The full-body image data, in DICOM format, was cropped to create a 3D bone geometry of the patient's left hand and visualized as an apparent hologram through the HoloLens (Figure 4.6).

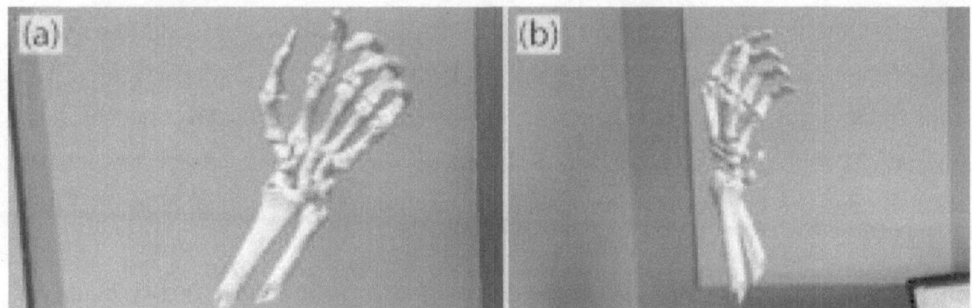

Figure 4.6: The 3D hand and wrist bone geometry visualized as a hologram in the real-world scene. (a) Anterior and (b) lateral view of 3D bone geometry as a virtual object.

4.4 Registering the AR visualization in situ – review of the literature

As stated in chapter 3 section 5, user calibration, fiducial marker and markerless tracking have been reported as solutions for registration in combination with AR medical systems. HoloLens AR medical literature that has implemented the three registration methods have been reviewed to determine the "Black Box" software and hardware modules used to solve the key processes identified in Chapter 3. The identified studies, as well as the assessment procedures used, are discussed below.

4.4.1 User calibration of the Microsoft HoloLens AR

The Novarad OpenSight system discussed in chapter 2 made use of the HoloLens and proprietary software to register the virtual object to the required surgical site automatically. However, if the registration was deemed inaccurate, the alignment was fine-tuned using manual calibration (hand gesture commands) (Gibby et al., 2018). A ruler was used to measure the perceived difference between the alignment of the virtual and real-world object after registration. Registration of the virtual object to the required location showed a circular deviation with the maximum average radius of the deviation as 2.5mm.

An intra-surgical HoloLens AR guidance system developed by Pratt et al. (2018) allowed for user calibration to register the visualization onto the surgical site. A polygon-based 3D volume rendering.OBJ file was used in an application developed in Unity 3D with components to allow for gesture and voice control. Pratt et al. (2018) assessed the time to align the virtual to real-world landmarks and found that making use of their HoloLens AR HMD system for intra-surgical navigation was less time-consuming than the current audible Doppler ultrasound navigation system being utilized. They did not present any quantitative registration accuracy assessment results, however, reported times between 1 and 2 minutes per registration.

Unity 3D (https://unity.com/) is a game engine developed by Unity Technologies and it supports all the major AR/VR platforms. To develop applications for the HoloLens, the Unity 3D Editor in combination with the Mixed Reality Toolkit (MRTK) for Unity is recommended (Rodrigues et al., 2017). The MRTK for Unity is an open-source GitHub (https://github.com/) repository project driven by Microsoft to help accelerate the development of applications for their Windows Mixed Reality devices. The prefabricated components and changes added to the Unity 3D editor by applying the MRTK Software development kit (SDK) settings to process the capturing of the real-world image footage, the determination of the FOV, and the required stereoscopic holographic rendering.

Vassallo et al. (2017) assessed the ability of the HoloLens to keep a virtual object stable at a defined point. The virtual object was placed in the real-world scene via the HoloLens native Holograms application. The pose of the virtual object was measured before and after the user walked away from and back to the virtual object. The respective pose of the virtual object was digitized through marking the perceived corners of the virtual object with the Polaris optical tracking system and a stylus with passive fiducial markers, before and after the spatial manipulation action. The Polaris optical tracking system is the most frequently used optical tracking system in IGS systems (Barfield, 2015), and makes use of both active and passive fiducial markers to determine the pose of the tracked object. The spatial stability of the Holograms application was also tested for sudden acceleration, occlusion, and object insertion during the experiments. Vassallo et al. (2017) stability assessment results of all four tests showed a mean error of 5.83mm with a standard deviation of 0.51mm in the pose of the virtual object after the influencing action had been performed.

4.4.2 Fiducial marker tracking with the Microsoft HoloLens AR

Andress et al. (2018) made use of the ARToolkit (https://github.com/artoolkit) open-source computer tracking library for the detection of a template marker, however, the game engine application platform was not specified. By adding the Vuforia SDK (https://developer.vuforia.com/) to Unity, Wu et al. (2018) developed a hybrid application that combined fiducial marker tracking and user calibration. Whilst wearing the HoloLens, a template marker (target image) was used to register the virtual object onto the real-world object, after which the user could manipulate the pose of the virtual object to solve for any perception errors. Wu et al., (2018) reported that the alignment errors where bounded within 3 mm. Compared to AR Toolkit, the Vuforia SDK can track the target image even if it is partially occluded as well as identify and track 3D images to allow for markerless tracking system development (PTC Inc., 2018).

El-Hariri et al. (2018) created a virtual object for Unity from a foam pelvis phantom with brass screws added into the surface of the pelvis model. The Vuforia SDK was used to align the virtual object with the real-world object when a custom-made target image was detected. Comparing the placement of virtual screws as seen through the HoloLens with the placement of the actual brass screws in the pelvis phantom, the total registration error could be established. The locations of the virtual and real-world screws were determined by marking the locations with a stylus, with passive fiducial markers, tracked by the Polaris optical tracking system. The study failed to specify the pose of the real and virtual objects in their respective XYZ Cartesian coordinate systems, yet reported a yielding root mean square error of 3.22mm in the x-direction, 22.46mm in the y-direction, and 28.30mm in the z-direction.

The Vuforia SDK is capable of recognizing and tracking the 2D planar target image even when it is wrapped around a cylinder as demonstrated by Frantz et al. (2018) who combined the HoloLens, Vuforia SDK version 6.5.22 and Unity version 2017.2.0f3. The study made use of a phantom skull as the real-world object, which was digitized to create the 3D virtual object. For the fiducial application, Vuforia's tarmac target image was used as the target image. The pose of the virtual object was defined in relation to the target image in the Unity application. A control application allowing for user calibration to register the virtual to real was developed to assess the performance of the fiducial tracking application. The registration of the virtual skull to the phantom skull was completed at a position of 0° and 80cm depth. Both the applications were tested for spatial alignment by marking the perceived location of the virtual object on a grid board attached to the bottom of the phantom skull. The perceived location of the virtual object was captured at -90°, -45°, 0°, 45° and 90°, with the applications reset between trails. For the user calibration application, a mean error in the alignment during the movements was reported as 4.39mm with a standard deviation of 1.29mm. Whereas, for the Vuforia built application a mean error of 1.41mm with a standard deviation 0.67mm was reported.

4.4.3 Markerless tracking with the Microsoft HoloLens AR

The HoloLens is a computer vision device and the camera modules on the HoloLens can be used to create a markerless registration system. Xie et al. (2017) developed a matching algorithm after 3D scanning the real-world object. Utilizing the surface mesh provided by the HoloLens's spatial mapping the pre-scanned surface point cloud could be matched to the real-world object to place the virtual object in the FOV, no results were detailed.

Making use of 3D scanning and matching algorithms for markerless registration could possibly lead to inaccuracies during intra-surgical guidance. The pose of the 3D scanned model would not match if the patient is moved to any other pose from the time of image modality capture (Pratt et al., 2018). The virtual object would also not necessarily match the real-world object if there is any tissue deformation (Zhang et al., 2019). And finally, making use of the HoloLens to track the patient's hand, could also deter from tracking the gesture movements made by the clinician to manipulate the AR visualization.

Consequently, a second optical tracking sensor could be used to locate the real-world object. Köhler (2017) combined the HoloLens with an optical motion tracker, the Leap Motion Controller (LMC), to develop more gesture-based interactions. Wang et al. (2017) combined the HoloLens and the LMC to create an AR telemedicine platform for remote procedural training. The FOV of the attending surgeon was augmented with visualizations of the remote surgeon's hands captured via the LMC. The LMC has also been used to assess and help rehabilitate the upper limb motor skills of Parkinson's disease patients (Butt et al., 2017). The LMC is a small motion sensor developed for gesture tracking of the hand (Figure 4.7). Leap Motion has made their Orion SDK available for open source project usage. The LMC's specifications are:

- 6.2mm thick, 25mm wide and 75mm long.
- 3 x infrared light-emitting diodes.
- 2 x monochromatic infra-red cameras.
- Universal serial bus 3 connectivity.

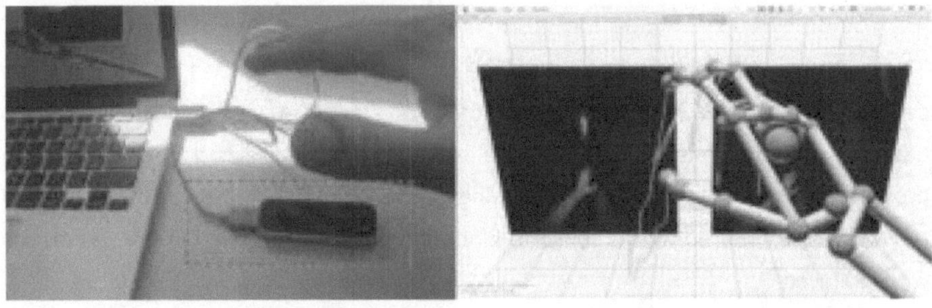

Figure 4.7: The Leap Motion Controller (red dashed rectangle in left image) is a tracking module specifically developed for tracking hand gestures.

4.5 Overview of the three AR HMD systems developed

The three registration methods discussed above have been used in combination with the HoloLens. The HoloLens (Figure 4.8) has the tracking modules, the video camera modules, the central processing unit, and the display models built into one complete unit. It can run the required software application untethered for spatial mapping, virtual object computing, image processing and rendering via the display module.

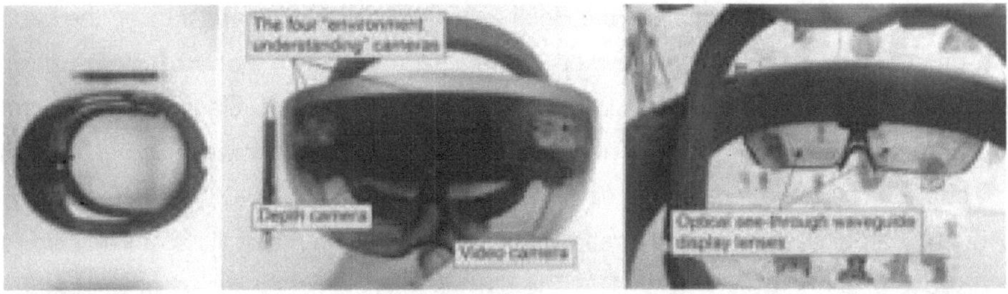

Figure 4.8: View of the Microsoft HoloLens's four "environment understanding" cameras, the time-of-flight depth camera sensor, and the optical see-through waveguide display lenses.

From the review of the literature, it emerged that the preferred software platform to develop the Black Box application at this point in time is the 3D game engine Unity in combination with the MRTK SDK. However, a mixture of SDKs and hardware assemblies is required for all three of the registration methods discussed. Therefore, in this project, three different AR HMD systems were developed to determine the best-suited method of registration for an AR HMD medical system. Each of the three prototype AR HMD systems developed consists of the HoloLens, Unity, and the MRTK SDK. All three AR HMD 3D game engine applications were developed using a personal distribution of Unity 2017.4.2f2 with the MRTK HoloToolkit-Unity-2017.4.2.0 GitHub repository imported as an asset.

To develop the user calibration AR HMD system (see chapter 6), only Unity and MTRK components were required in combination with the HoloLens. To create a fiducial marker tracking system, the developed AR HMD system combined the Vuforia SDK, a target image, the HoloLens, Unity, and the MRTK SDK (chapter 7). To create the markerless tracking AR HMD system (chapter 8), the LMC was added. Leap Motion's Orion SDK was combined with the MRTK SDK in Unity to enable tracking of the 3D printed hand.

Experiments were designed to assess which of the registration protocols would be best suited to develop the intra-surgical guidance AR HMD medical system. The experimental parameters and procedures are detailed in the following sections.

4.6 Dependent and independent variables

When validating an AR medical system, the analysis can be completed through both quantitative and qualitative approaches to experimentation. Quantitative analysis entails testing the functional performance of the system, whereas qualitative analysis assesses the user interaction of the developed AR function or system (Barsom et al., 2016). The three developed AR HDM systems were analysed to produce quantifiable results. User calibration was assessed for the first AR HMD system. Fiducial market tracking was assessed for the second AR HMD system. Markerless tracking was assessed for the third AR HMD system.

Generating quantifiable experiments requires identifying the dependent and independent variables of the hypothesis. A dependent variable is a measured fact, i.e. the cause and effect of the hypothesis. Any measurement or changes completed on the dependent variable will influence the outcome of the experiment. The independent variables are the properties that influence the dependent variable and can be manipulated or altered independently. Normally the independent variables are the controlled factors in an experiment to test the cause and effect of a specified hypothesis on the dependent variables. For the use case of intra-surgical guidance, the required simulation is the viewing of the virtual object as a holographic AR visualization, at the required location as specified by the user (clinician), for example, the surgical site. To discern the best performing AR HMD system to fulfil the required task, the dependent variables are:

1. The registration accuracy of the virtual object to the required position (measured in millimetres).
2. The spatial alignment (spatial registration) accuracy of the virtual object to the required surgical location in 3D space.
3. The spatial stability of the system. In other words, the ability of the AR HMD system to keep the 3D virtual object anchored to the required location.
4. The frames per second (fps) rendering capability of the AR medical system (measured in fps). If the rendering frame rate is too low the clinician will see the re-rendering of the virtual object, which would distract the clinician from the usefulness of the AR medical system.

To gauge the above-mentioned dependent variables, several independent variables can be identified. Firstly, the registration method used, in this case, 1) user calibration, 2) fiducial marker tracking, or 3) markerless tracking, to align the Cartesian coordinate system of the virtual object to the required real-world location's Cartesian coordinate system. Secondly, user-specific independent variables such as the movement of the clinician around the surgical site (specifically, after the AR view has been created), the angle of the observation, the height of the clinician, or the quality of the clinician's eyesight and perception of the virtual object. Environment-specific variables such as the lighting conditions or a change in the spatial environment (spatial mapping variables) can also be regarded as independent variables, for example, the introduction of new equipment or movement of the patient whilst keeping the required real-world point of visualization constant. Independent variables can also include key performance metrics such as the file size of the virtual object, or the rendering quality of the computer-generated visual image. In this and the following sections, for the purposes of experimentation, the required real word location has been represented as a real-world object matching the virtual object. As such, the required location is referred to as the real-world object hereafter.

4.7 Assessment parameters

For the purpose of assessing the capabilities of the three AR HMD systems, the following dependent variables were identified to be evaluated: 1) The accuracy of the initial registration of the AR HMD system before applying the relevant registration method. 2) The virtual object's spatial registration accuracy based on a simulation of movement of the clinician around the surgical site and 3) the spatial stability of the AR HMD system: the extent to which the virtual object is kept in the same place during multiple movements of the clinician. As stated previously, inaccurate registration could mislead the clinician and cause grave harm. However, the required accuracy of the registration is determined by the intervention performed. In general, for IGS procedures, an accuracy of 1 to 2 mm is considered acceptable (Meulstee et al., 2019). As such, 2mm was set as the benchmark for the initial alignment accuracy. The initial alignment accuracy of the AR HMD systems and corresponding registration protocols were measured after applying one of the registration methods and placing the HoloLens a 100cm away from the rear of the real-world object at point P_A as shown in Figure 4.9.

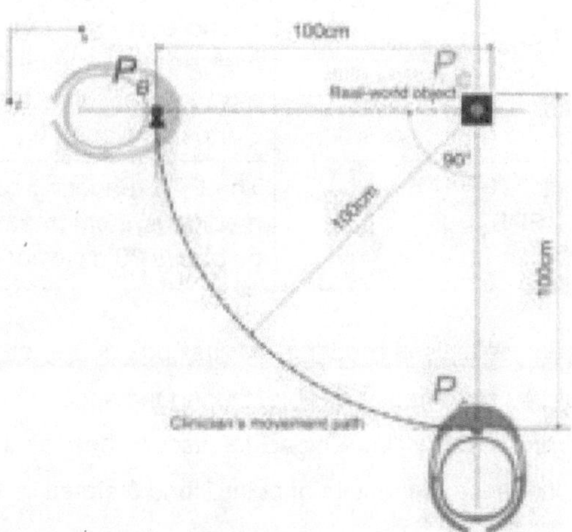

Figure 4.9: Depiction of the initial alignment position of the Microsoft HoloLens to the real-world object and the simulated clinician movement path.

To examine the spatial alignment variable, a clinician's movement was simulated as a clockwise movement from 0° (Point P_A) to 90° (Point P_B) with a movement radius of 100cm from the real-world object (Point P_C) in the XZ plane (see Figure 4.9). To assess the spatial stability, a second movement following the same path was completed from P_B to P_A, and back to P_B. As the virtual object needs to stay at the specified location, 2mm tolerance was also considered as the benchmarking value for the spatial alignment and spatial stability. To summarise, the quantitative experimental parameters are detailed in Table 4.3 below.

Table 4.3: The quantitative experimental assessment parameters

Nr.	Parameter	Assessment description
1	Initial registration accuracy	The accuracy during initial alignment of the virtual object to the required position at point P_A in the XY plane (required to be 2mm at any point).
2	Spatial alignment	The spatial alignment of the virtual object after the clinician had moved through 90° at a radius of 100cm around the required position (required to be 2mm at any point in the ZY plane).
3	Spatial stability	The spatial stability of the AR HMD system to keep the 3D virtual object anchored to the required position with multiple movements (set to be 2mm at any point in the corresponding Cartesian plane).
4	FPS	The FPS rendering capability of the AR medical system (measured in fps) must be above 30fps to not see the rendering.

Two procedures were established, during the first procedure, all other independent variables were kept as constant as possible. During the second procedure, a change in the spatial environment was introduced to discern how changes in the spatial environment might influence the results of point 2 and 3 stated in Table 4.3.

4.8 Materials and setup

To quantitatively evaluate the accuracy of registration, spatial alignment, and spatial stability, a computer-generated 3D cube was used (Figure 4.10 (a)). The rationale was that a regular shape of known dimensions would facilitate for a more accurate and precise assessment of registration accuracy, spatial alignment, and spatial stability, than an irregular object such as the hand. Any inaccuracy and imprecision detection using the cube would translate to more complex shapes. The 3D cube, size 50x50x50mm, was created in Autodesk Inventor (2018) and 3D printed using a Zortax M200 3D printer. A plinth was fabricated to house the real-world object(s) at position P_C and was attached to a tripod as shown by Figure 4.10 (b), the combined view of the virtual 3D cube and the 3D printed cube captured via Microsoft's Mixed Reality Capture (MRC).

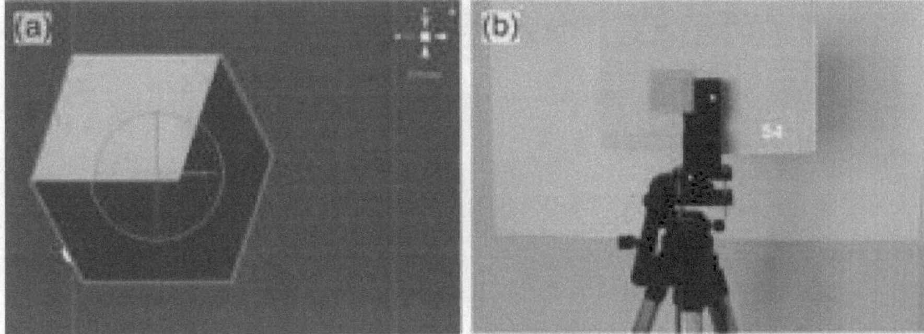

Figure 4.10: The irregular shaped 3D anatomically hand model was substituted with a 3D cube to allow for assessment of registration parameters (a) The simplified 3D cube geometry in the Unity scene. (b) The virtual 3D cube and the 3D printed cube combined in the FOV via the Microsoft HoloLens.

The plinth and tripod combination (henceforth referred to as a rig) was fabricated to hold either of the 3D printed real-world object (s) and a grid board (Figure 4.11 (a)). The 3D real-world object supporting rig was fabricated to allow the interchanging of the real-world objects (Figure 4.11 (b)). The grid board was an A4 hardboard with grid paper; the grid paper had 5 mm spacing major lines only. The grid board was used to measure any possible errors in registration between virtual and real as well as to calculate scaling factors for measurements (See Appendix A section 4).

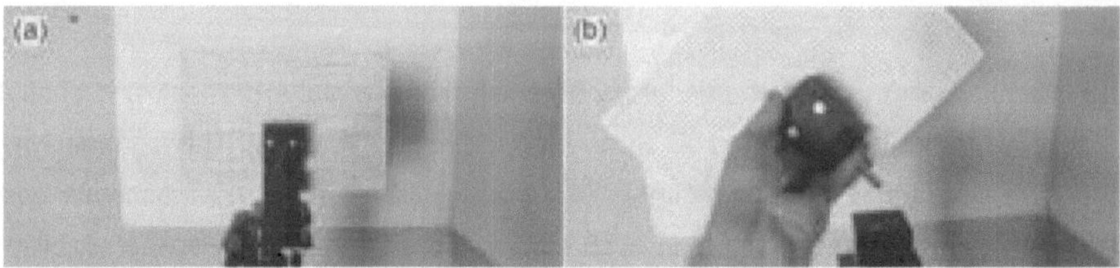

Figure 4.11: Rig P_C assembly (a) The 3D printed cube could easily be combined with the grid board to form the P_C rig (b) The 3D printed cube and hand were fabricated to allow for interchanging of the real-world objects.

Two more plinths were fabricated to support the HoloLens at position P_A and P_B to be combined with a tripod each (Figure 4.12 (a)) which could be set to a maximum height of 150cm. As such, the heights of all three the rigs were all set to 150cm from the floor. This was completed by setting the heights of the rigs to a mark made 150cm from the floor on one of the test area's walls (Figure 4.12 (b)).

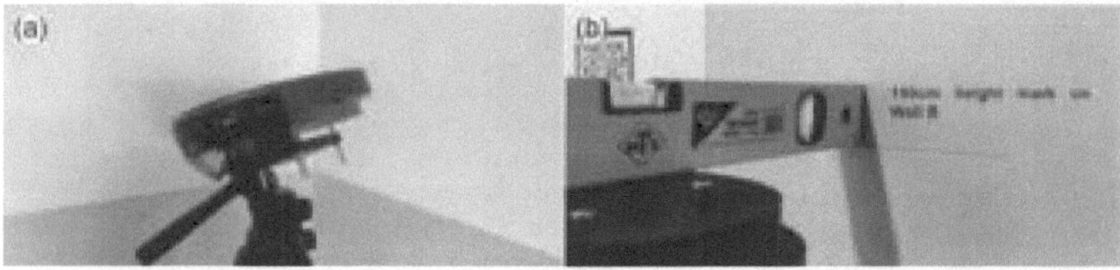

Figure 4.12: HoloLens supporting rig assembly and height calibration of the rigs. (a) Photo of one of the two Microsoft HoloLens rigs assembled. (b) The height of the rigs was set to 150cm using a mark on one of the test area's walls (Wall B).

The three rigs were used to arrange the HoloLens and the real-world object(s) in the test area. All the materials and equipment required for the experiments are listed in Table 4.4, and Figure 4.13 below illustrates the test area as a layout schematic of the materials to match the arrangement specified in Figure 4.9. Items no. 13 to 17 were used to calibrate the setup and ensure reproducibility. As stated, P_A was the starting point (0°), and P_B (90°) the point to which the HoloLens would be moved to simulate a clinician's movement. In the schematic P_A and P_B represent the locations of the two HoloLens rigs, and P_C the location of the real-world object with gird board rig.

Table 4.4: Specification of materials and equipment used for experimental procedures.

Item no.	Description	Quantity	Nomenclature in Figure 4.12
1	Tripod (Mivision 5858D) for Position A with 3D printed HoloLens plinths - Mivision 5858D	1	P_A rig
2	Tripod (Mivision 5858D) for Position B with 3D printed HoloLens plinths	1	P_B rig
3	3D printed cube	1	Part of the P_C rig
4	3D printed hand (the skin layer)	1	Not in schematic
5	Tripod for Position C with 3D printed plinth to hold the 3D printed cube and the Leap Motion.	1	P_C rig
6	An A4 hardboard with grid paper, with major lines only, 5 mm spacing.	2	Grid board
7	A 50x120mm hardboard with the template marker.	1	Target image
8	Microsoft HoloLens Gen 1	1	HoloLens
9	Leap Motion + USB cable	1	Leap
10	Tenda AC6 Smart 11AC Dual-Band Wi-Fi Router	1	Tenda AP
11	Razer Blade Stealth 13"	1	Razer
12	The Huawei B593 LTE router	1	Not in Figure 4.12
13	Measuring tape	2	Not in Figure 4.12
14	Fabricated meter stick, length 180cm	2	Not in Figure 4.12
15	Spirit level	2	Not in Figure 4.12
16	Protractor	1	Not in Figure 4.12
17	Double-sided tape to fix tripods to floor	1	Not in Figure 4.12

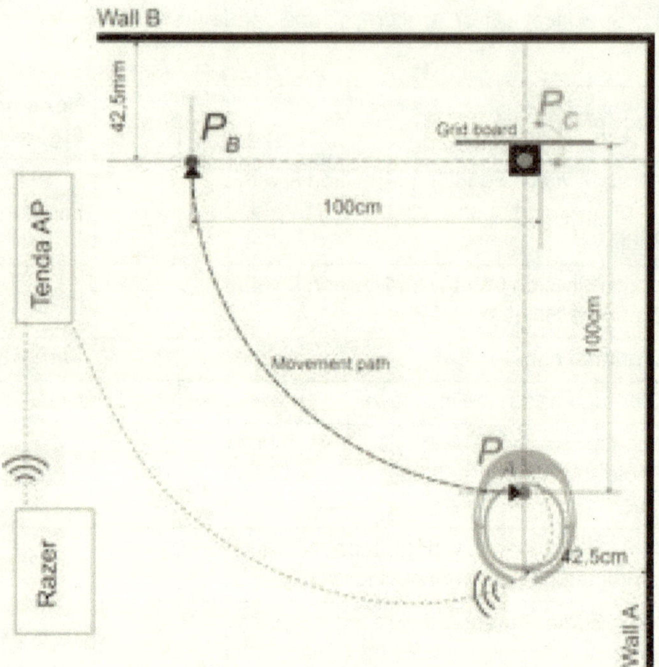

Figure 4.13: Layout schematic of the test area showing the required position of the AR HMD medical system components (not to scale)

An assumed position of the HoloLens's centre (origin of FOV) was used to calibrate the location of the HoloLens from the rear of the real-world cube at P_C, as no technical data could be identified detailing the HoloLens's centre of origin (see Figure 4.14 (a)). The rationale for this assumption was the strap of the HoloLens would be resting against the user's forehead at this point, similar to the point on the HoloLens plinth depicted in Figure 4.14 (b).

To achieve the layout schematic, the identified points on the HoloLens plinths were used in combination with fabricated meter sticks to place rig A (P_A) and rig B (P_B) 100cm away from the rear of the real-world object located at P_C (Figure 4.14 (c) and (d)). The centres of the P_A, P_B, and P_C rigs were aligned and placed at right angles to each other. The combined components and equipment are referred to as the test rig with the real-world Cartesian coordinate system **W**.

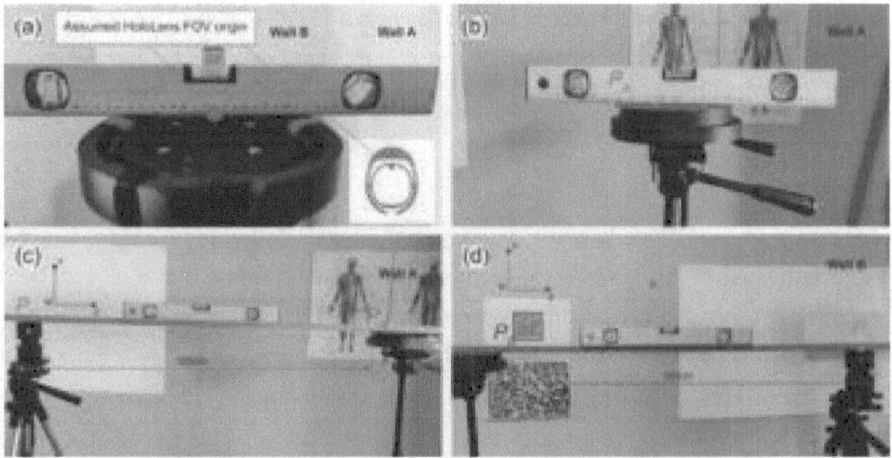

Figure 4.14: Calibration of the test area and rigs. (a)The location of the HoloLens's centre (origin of FOV) was assumed at the place where the strap would be attached. (b) The HoloLens plinths and angular alignment were checked for all the rigs using a spirit level. (c) and (d) Fabricated meter sticks were used to place rig A (P_A) and rig B (P_B) a 100cm away from the rear of the real-world object located at P_C.

4.9 Simulation of clinician movement

Two procedures were used to simulate the movement of the clinician around the real and virtual objects, an assumption was made that the user (clinician) would be standing and would be required to move around the patient, the real-world object. The differences between the two procedures are discussed below.

4.9.1 First simulation: Clinician movement with no change in the spatial environment prior to movement.

During the first simulation, the HoloLens was moved from P_A to P_B clockwise, before the grid board was rotated at P_C. The grid board was rotated by lifting the combined real-world cube and grid board out of the rig at P_C and rotating it by 90° to face P_B to allow the capture of misalignment. The HoloLens was then moved back to P_A counter-clockwise, the real cube and gird board rotated, and the process repeated. This procedure aimed to simulate a spatial environment that stays the same before and during movement of the HoloLens around the real and virtual object, i.e. the clinician moving around a still patient onto which the virtual patient data has been registered.

4.9.2 Second simulation: Change in the spatial environment before moving around the real-world object

During the second procedure, the grid board at P_C was rotated to face P_B before the HoloLens was moved from P_A to P_B through 90°. The movement of the grid board explored a change in the spatial environment before the movement of the HoloLens around the real-world object. Theoretically, the HoloLens should update the spatial map created to allow for any changes in the real environment.

4.9.3 The trials

For each AR HMD system assessment, three trials of both the procedures were completed to test for random occurrence or patterns in the results. The three Unity built registration applications were closed and launched after each trial to ensure a cold-start, thus removing any spatial mapping data that was captured during the previous trial; so as not to affect future trials.

4.10 Calibration and assessment of the AR HMD systems

The interpupillary distance was calibrated using the native Calibration Application (part of the HoloLens suite) only once. Calibrations to ensure the performance of the three AR HMD system applications preceded the experiments. The CPU and GPU loads were reduced by setting the stereoscopic rendering method to a single pass instance with the quality of the graphics to be rendered set to "High" instead of "Ultra" in Unity. Normally, these settings are determined by the requirements of the application, but for coherence, they were set to the same values for all three of the applications. The depth buffering feature in Unity was enabled for better hologram stability as recommended by Microsoft. With the feature enabled, the spatial map produced during the application is shared with the Windows Mixed Reality platform to better optimize hologram stability for any given frame being rendered by the application. The Unity built applications were deployed to the HoloLens via Visual Studio (2017), as required.

Microsoft's Mixed Reality Capture (MRC) feature was used to capture the pose of the virtual object in the real environment at the key positions to assess the accuracy of registration, the spatial alignment, and the spatial stability of the three AR HMD systems. Mixed reality capture allows the capturing of the FOV in real-time, from the perspective of the HoloLens, by means of a video recording or a photograph. Mixed Reality Capture can be natively accessed on the HoloLens or remotely via the Windows Device Portal. With the use of MRC, the user-specific independent variables, such as the angle of the observation, the height of the clinician, and perception of the virtual object, are circumvented as detailed in chapter 4 section 6. The qualitative assessment of what or how the virtual object is perceived by the user versus what has been captured by the MRC photo did not form part of the scope of work completed for this study.

It should be noted that the setup and list of components had to change slightly for each of the AR HMD systems. Each of the AR HMD systems required a different set of SDKs, software settings, and hardware components to achieve the specified registration method and virtual object visualization in the FOV via the HoloLens. The system architecture required, and the corresponding assessment of the AR HMD systems are detailed in the ensuing chapters. As the AR HMD systems had to change to allow for the different registration protocols, so to the sequence of mixed reality photos captured to document the pose of the virtual object in the real-world environment. For clarity, the structure of the ensuing chapters follows the format below:

1. A description of the relevant AR HMD system's architecture and feasibility analysis with the 3D virtual and printed hand models.
2. A description of the setup for quantitative analysis of the AR HMD system.
3. The procedures and the sequence of MRC photos (the full complement of captured photos are in Appendix A).

The processed results of the quantitative analysis and discussion of the measured variable

Chapter 5: User calibration for virtual object registration with an AR HMD system

The Jux3DModel AR HMD system was developed to assess a user calibration approach to registering the virtual objects to real-world objects with the Microsoft HoloLens.

5.1 The Jux3DModel AR HMD system

The Mixed Reality Toolkit (MRTK) SDK was utilised for the development of the Unity application for the Jux3DModel AR HMD system. Both the simplified 3D arm volume and the 3D cube were imported as assets to Unity and added as Game Objects in the scene hierarchy structure. The notable MRTK components and relevant settings that were implemented are discussed in Table 5.1, with the system architecture of the Jux3DModel AR HMD system detailed in Figure 5.1.

Table 5.1: Notable MRTK components used.

MRTK component	Description of use
MixedRealityCameraParent assembly prefab	Takes care of FOV tracking and stereoscopic rendering
SpatialMapping prefab	Maps the real world as a virtual mesh at specified time intervals. The time between spatial mapping updates was set to a default of 3.5 seconds and 500 triangles per cubic meter.
InputManager prefab	Follows the line of sight of the user to detect gesture input.
TwoHandManipulatable C# script	Allows for manipulating objects with one or two hands and was applied to the Game Objects to enable the "Air tap" gesture.
FPS Display prefab	Prefab that allows for the capture of the fps rendering capabilities. The FPS Display prefab was added to the Unity scene hierarchy and configured with the TapToPlace component to trigger a request to update the spatial map already captured; it also aided in obtaining the fps measurement.
TapToPlace C# script	C# script that calls to action SpatialMapping.

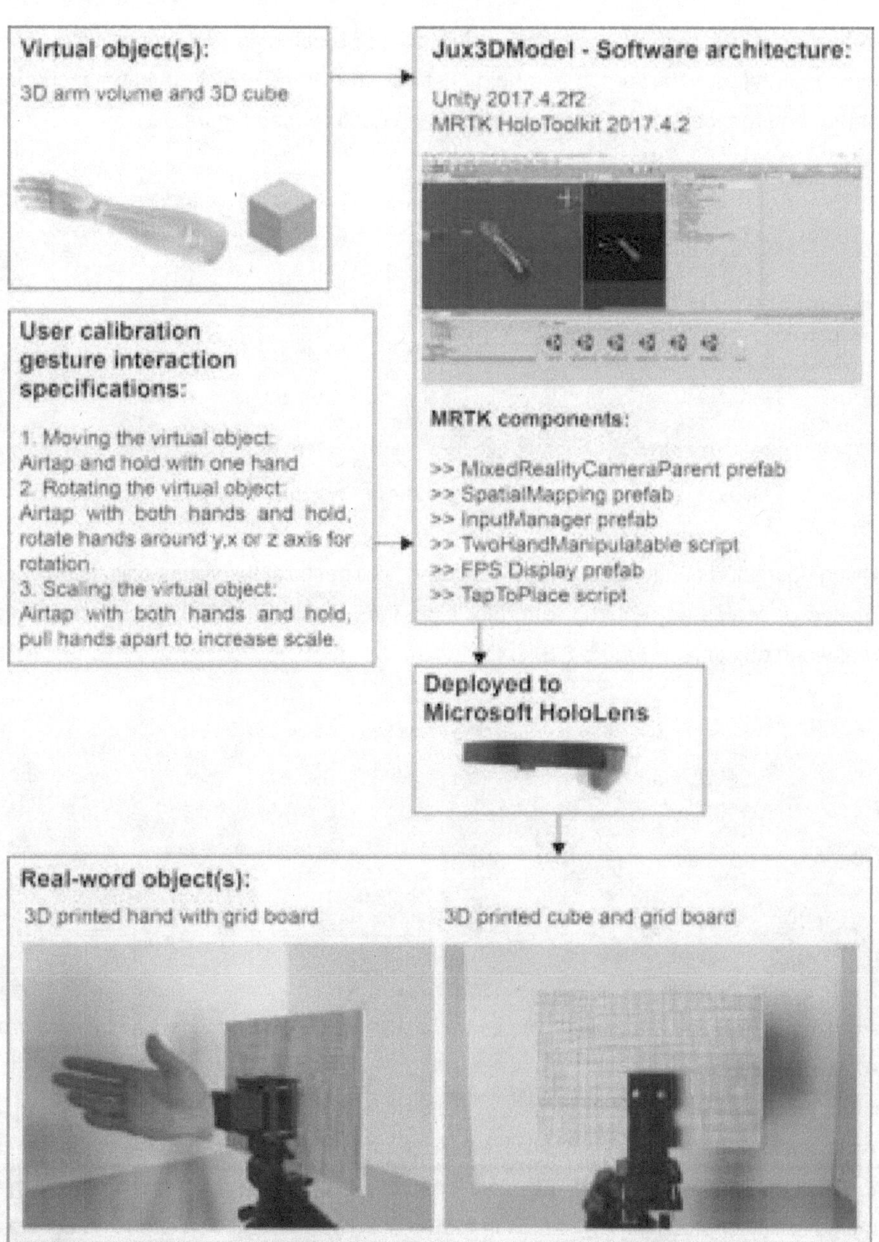

Figure 5.1: Process flow of the Jux3DModel AR HMD system to assess virtual to real-world object registration via user calibration.

With the Air tap gesture, the virtual object could be selected and moved using one hand orientated in the Air tap and hold gesture. The virtual object could be anchored at the required location by releasing the Air tap gesture (see Figure 5.2).

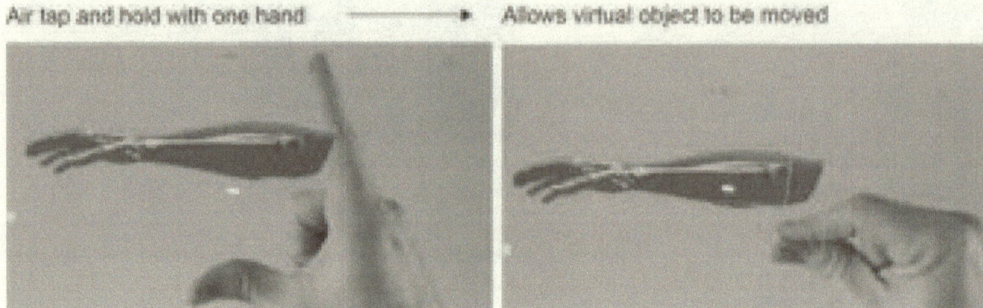

Figure 5.2: Moving the virtual object with the Air tap gesture to enable user calibration.

Using both hands orientated in the Air tap and hold gesture, the virtual object could be rotated or scaled as required to further align the virtual object to the corresponding real-world object (see Figure 5.3).

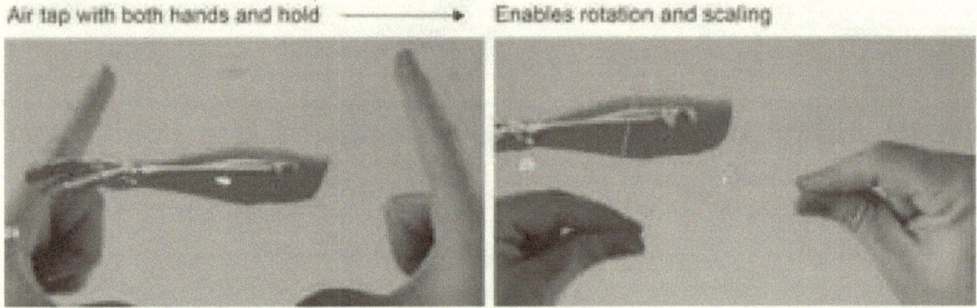

Figure 5.3: Rotating and scaling the virtual object with the two-handed Air tap gesture to enable user calibration.

As shown in Figure 5.4 (a) it is feasible to align the AR visualization of the virtual hand to its 3D printed counterpart with user calibration. Unfortunately, as shown by the mixed reality capture (MRC) photos in Figure 5.4 (b), when the real-world object was moved, the alignment was lost. This is akin to the real-world need to be solved, namely patients moving after initial registration, which results in a re-registration required (see chapter 2 section 8.4).

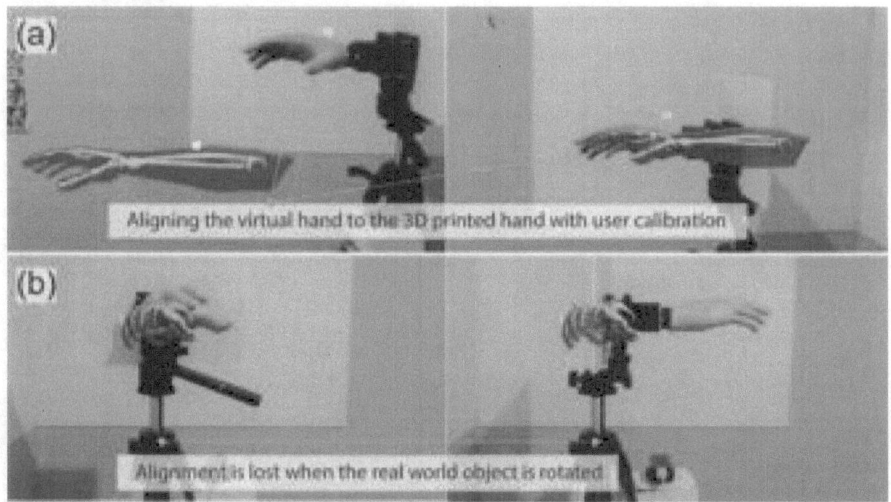

Figure 5.4: FOV whilst wearing the Microsoft HoloLens recorded with MRC to practically explore whether user calibration can be used to align the virtual hand to the 3D printed hand. (a) Alignment of the 3D virtual hand to the 3D printed hand. (b) Alignment lost due to rotating the 3D printed hand.

5.2 Jux3DModel AR HMD system assessment

In the Unity virtual scene (Cartesian coordinate system **V**) the distance of the virtual cube from the centre of origin of the MixedRealityCamera prefab was set to match the real-world environment's test rig setup - a 100cm distance from the back of the virtual cube in the XZ plane to the centre of origin (depicted in Figure 5.5). The centre line of the virtual cube was placed 25mm to the left of the MixedRealityCamera's centreline in the XY plane to allow for distinguishing between the virtual and real cube (Cartesian coordinate system **R**) in the MRC photo captured at the launch of the Jux3DModel AR HMD system. The 25mm XY plane setting would be removed when the user wears the HoloLens to align the virtual object to the real-world object during user calibration. The Jux3DModel Unity built application was deployed to the HoloLens via Visual Studio and launched with the HoloLens placed on the P_A rig. The sequence of MRC photos captured is detailed in Table 5.2. Figure 5.6 and Figure 5.7 depict the flow of the two procedures used to evaluate user calibration as a method for registration via the Jux3Model AR HMD system. For both procedures, three trials were recorded.

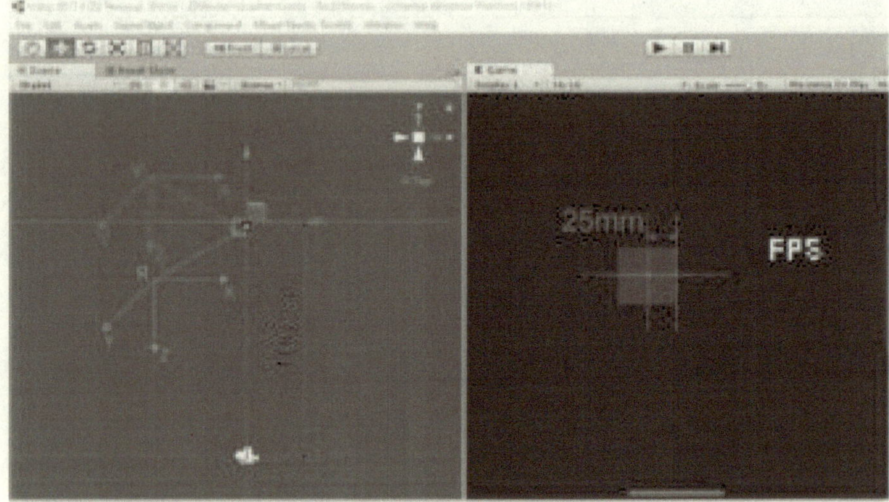

*Figure 5.5: The corresponding measurements between the real-world object centre point **R** and the virtual object centre point **V** for the development of the Jux3Dmodel Unity application.*

Table 5.2: Sequence of MRC photos captured during the Jux3Dmodel AR HMD system assessment.

Description	MRC Photo (Abbreviation)
MRC photo captured after the HoloLens was placed at P_A of the launch of the Jux3DModel application.	P_{LA}
MRC photo captured after the HoloLens was moved through 90° clockwise to P_B.	P_{LB}
MRC photo captured after the HoloLens was moved back close to P_A, "Air tap" user calibration used to align the virtual to the real-world cube.	P_{UA}
MRC photo captured for the assessment of user calibration registration alignment at P_A.	P_{A1}
MRC photo captured after the HoloLens was moved through 90° clockwise to assess spatial alignment at P_B.	P_{B1}
MRC photo captured after the HoloLens was moved back to P_A to assess spatial stability at P_A.	P_{A2}
MRC photo captured after the HoloLens was moved back to P_B to assess spatial stability at P_B.	P_{B2}

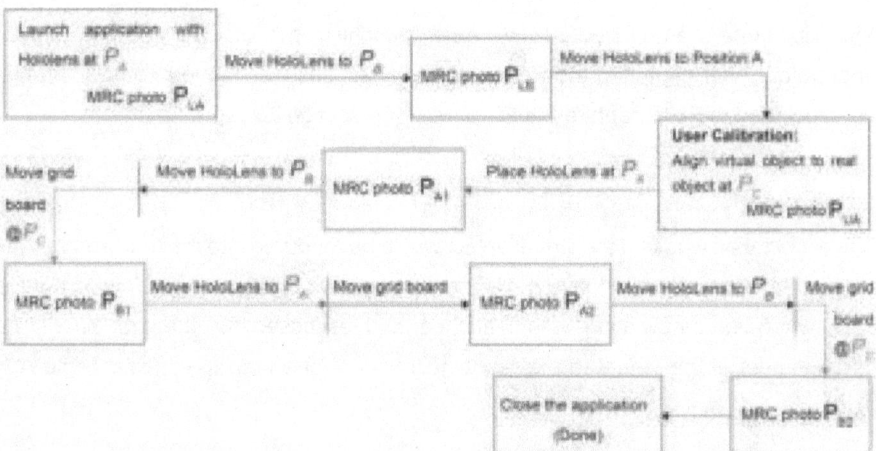

Figure 5.6: Procedure 1 process flow to simulate a stable spatial environment during the Jux3DModel trails.

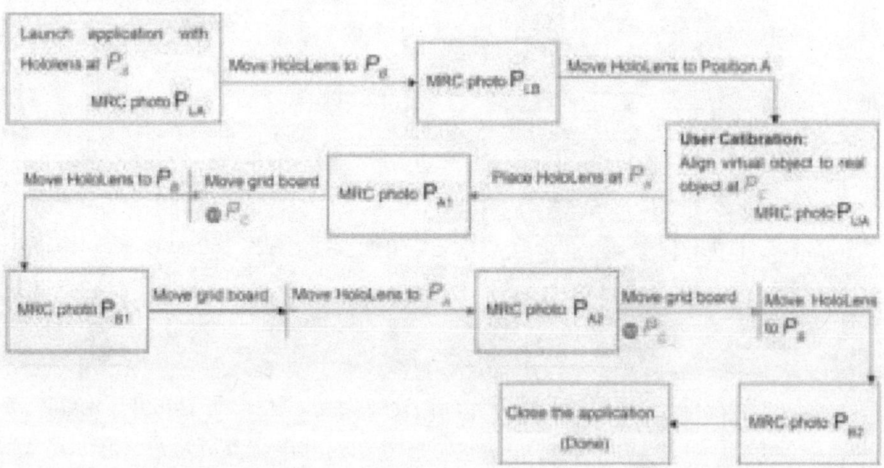

Figure 5.7: Procedure 2 process flow to simulate a changing spatial environment during the Jux3DModel trails and track capturing of MRC photos.

5.3 Registration accuracy at P_A in the XY plane

The HoloLens was placed at PA after launching the Jux3DModel's deployed application. After capturing the P_{LA} photo, the HoloLens was moved from P_A through 90° clockwise to P_B to capture the P_{LB} photo (see section 7.5).

5.3.1 Alignment at the launch of the AR HMD System at P_A

The expectation was that the virtual object would be rendered into the real-world scene according to the calibrated layout. However, as shown in Figure 5.8 this was not the case when the application was launched and assessed for the first time. The misalignment of the virtual to the real object varied for all the trials (See Table A.1, Appendix A.1).

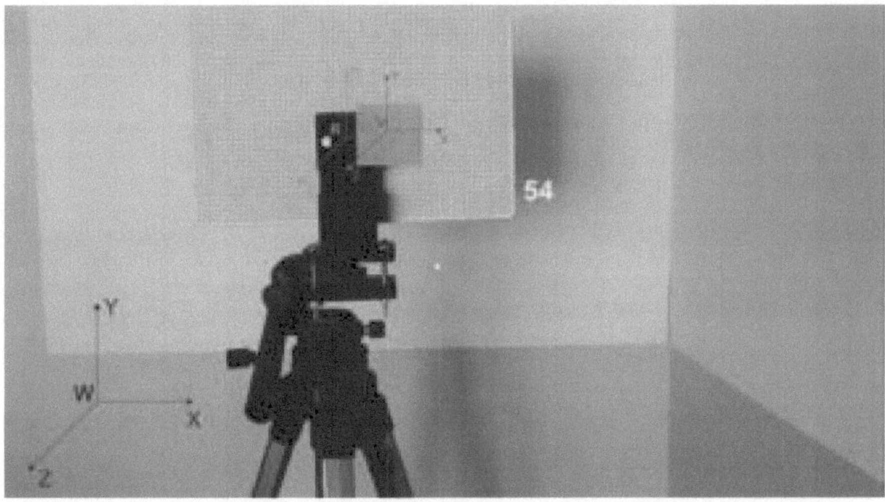

Figure 5.8: The MRC P_{LA} photo showing the misalignment of the virtual to real-world cube detected after the launch of the Jux3Dmodel application during procedure 1 trial 1.

5.3.2 Registration accuracy after user calibration registration

After the capture of the P_{LB} photo, the HoloLens was moved counter-clockwise back towards P_A. User calibration was completed while the author wore the HoloLens, before placement of the HoloLens on the P_A rig, and recorded with the capture of the

MRC photo P_{UA} for all trials. The height of the HoloLens, when worn from the floor, was 175cm with the author standing next to the P_{A} rig. To assess the accuracy of the user calibration, the HoloLens was moved vertically through 25cm and placed on the P_{A} rig. At this point, the XZ plane of the virtual and real-world objects would not be visible, and the registration alignment was captured via the MRC P_{A1} photo. To quantitatively calculate the registration accuracy of the Jux3Dmodel AR HMD system, the Euclidean distance between the top left corners of the real and virtual cube was measured in the XY plane using the P_{A1} photo. The Euclidean distance errors between the top left corners of the real and virtual cube ranged from 6.773mm (Figure 5.9 (a) to 20.809mm (Figure 5.9 (b)). The arrows detail the resultant direction of the vector in the figures. The Euclidian distance errors of all the trials with all relevant x- and y-axis displacements are reported in Table 5.3.

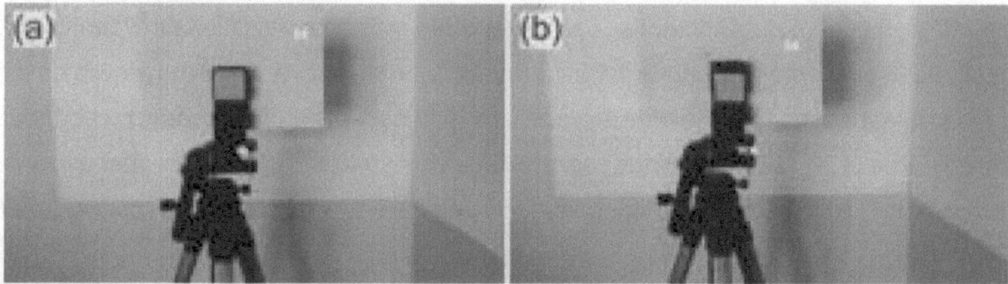

Figure 5.9: Assessment of registration errors identified in the MRC P_{A1} photos. (a) P_{A1} of procedure 1 trial 1. (b) P_{A1} of procedure 2 trial 3.

Table 5.3: Difference in position between the top left corners of the real cube and the virtual cube at P_{A1} measured in the XY plane.

Description	Euclidian distance error (mm)	Y-axis displacement error (mm)	X-axis displacement error (mm)
Procedure 1 Trial 1	6.7773	-5.553	3.858
Procedure 1 Trial 2	15.176	-13.346	7.217
Procedure 1 Trial 3	14.010	-13.267	4.484
Procedure 2 Trial 1	19.985	-17.008	10.515
Procedure 2 Trial 2	18.988	-17.273	7.886
Procedure 2 Trial 3	20.809	-19.478	7.311

5.3.3 Discussion of the initial alignment results

Point-to-point registration normally refers to the process of matching the point cloud structures of two similar virtual objects. By calibrating the virtual scene to match the real-world scene, the setup of the Jux3DModel AR HMD system could have been described as a virtual point to real-world point registration method. The error in the alignment at the launch of the Jux3DModel AR HMD system can be attributed to the inaccurate angular calibration of the HoloLens on the P_A rig in the XZ plane. This observation was confirmed by the varying locations of the virtual cube in the P_{LA} photos during the repeated trials.

Frantz et al. (2018) reported a registration alignment error of 0.62mm at 0° for their control application discussed in chapter 5 section 4.2. However, the surface point localisation in the control condition showed a mean error of 5.43mm. With regard to registration alignment, Gibby et al. (2018) reported a circular deviation between virtual and real-world objects, with a mean error of 2.5mm and a standard deviation of 0.44mm. However, the HoloLens's position in those experiments never changed. Finally, Rae et al. (2018) reported registration errors smaller than 10mm, after aligning holographic fiducial markers to corresponding real-world landmarks during user calibration.

It is in the opinion of the author that with enough practice, a clinician might be able to reach the required 2mm or less accuracy alignment of the entire virtual objects pose. However, the alignment errors in the P_{A1} photos are of a much larger scale and makes the use of the Jux3DModel application unfit for intra-surgical guidance at this time as the clinician will have to move and with the shown virtual object drift user calibration re-alignment will continuously be required. The notable drift identified resulted in the Jux3DModel AR HMD system performing worse than any of the published studies reviewed. The drift also followed a pattern of a negative change in the Y-axis and positive in the X-axis, thus following the movement of the HoloLens as it was moved from the authors head and placed on the P_A rig.

5.4 Spatial alignment accuracy at P_B

As detailed in the procedure flows (Figure 5.6 and Figure 5.7), the HoloLens was moved from P_A through 90° clockwise to P_B with the real cube and grid board rotated accordingly to face P_B thereafter. The movement from P_A to P_B was repeated three times with user calibration initiated during the first movement from P_B back to P_A.

5.4.1 Spatial alignment at the launch of the AR HMD System P_B

The MRC P_{LB} photos were captured to determine whether the calibrated spatial alignment between the virtual and real-world scenes matched. A misalignment between the real and virtual object centres in the YZ-plane was identified in the P_{LB} photos for all the trials (Figure 5.10). The magnitude of the misalignment error in the P_{LB} photos had a mean distance of 75.62mm between the real and virtual centres of the cubes with a standard deviation of 3.23mm. For a detailed calculation of the mean and standard deviation see Table A.9, Appendix A.4.

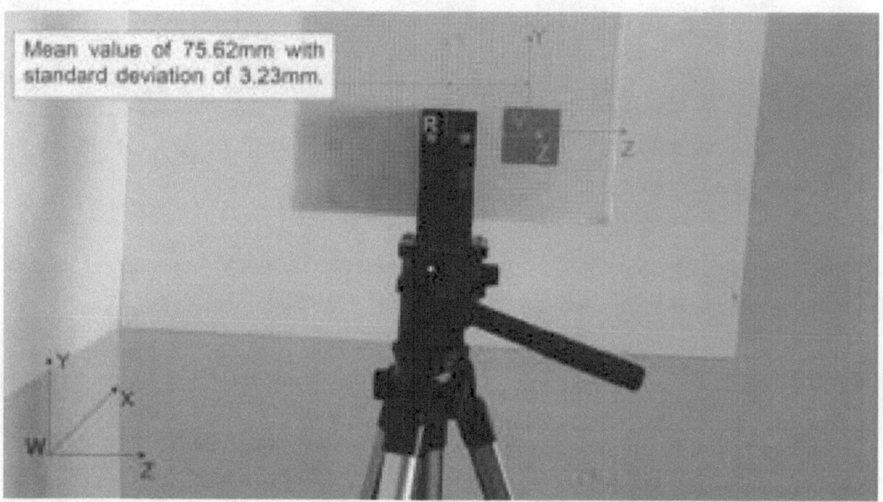

Figure 5.10: MRC P_{LB} photo showing the mean spatial misalignment error of the virtual to the real-world cube.

5.4.2 Spatial alignment accuracy after user calibration registration

To measure the spatial alignment the HoloLens was moved back to P_B and placed on the P_B rig. For procedure 1 the grid board was rotated after this movement whilst for procedure 2, the grid board rotation preceded the movement of the HoloLens. The spatial alignment results are identified in the MRC P_{B1} photos of both procedures. To calculate the spatial alignment accuracy the Euclidean distance between the top left corners of the real and virtual cube identified in the P_{A1} photo was measured in the YZ plane using the corresponding procedures P_{B1} photo. The Euclidean distance between the top left corners of the real and virtual cubes as identified in P_{B1} ranged from 85.456mm (Figure 5.11(a)) to 166.156mm (Figure 5.11(b)). The relevant displacement errors identified for all of the trials are reported in Table 5.4.

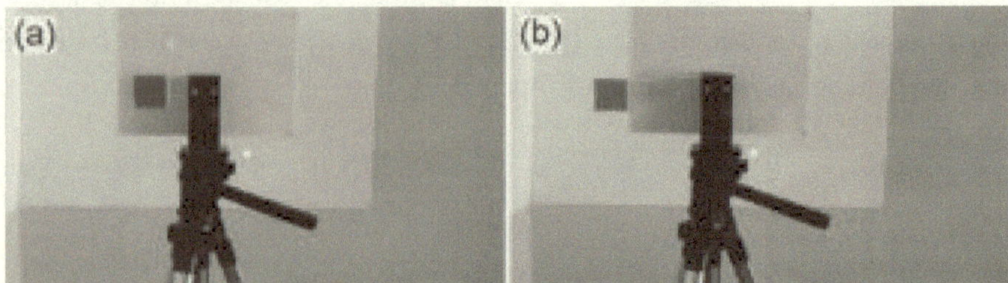

Figure 5.11: Spatial alignment errors identified in the MRC P_{B1} photos. (a) P_{B1} of procedure 1 trial 2. (b) P_{B1} of procedure 2 trial 1.

Table 5.4: Absolute difference in position between the top left corners of the real cube and the virtual cube at P_{B1} (the top right corner in the YZ plane pictures).

Description	**Euclidian distance error (mm)**	**Y-axis displacement error (mm)**	**Z-axis displacement error (mm)**
Procedure 1 Trial 1	85.456	-16.694	-85.437
Procedure 1 Trial 2	94.269	-9.393	-93.793
Procedure 1 Trial 3	80.392	-10.571	-79.696
Procedure 2 Trial 1	166.156	-9.457	-165.878
Procedure 2 Trial 2	163.483	-11.067	-163.119
Procedure 2 Trial 3	136.168	-13.324	-135.508

5.4.3 Discussion of the spatial alignment results

The spatial misalignment in the P_{LB} photos cannot be attributed to the angular calibration error in the XZ-plane of the HoloLens on the P_A rig due to the substantial mean error and standard deviation identified. The error could possibly be attributed to the difference of the assumed centre of origin point vs the real centre of origin of the HoloLens in the z-direction. However, this would need to be analysed further on a more precise rig to determine the exact position of the HoloLens's centre of origin. The misalignment errors in the P_{A1} and P_{B1} photos speaks to an inherent drift error in spatial capabilities of the Jux3DModel AR HMD system in 3D, with the drift again following the direction of the movement of the HoloLens.

For comparison, the performance of the control application developed by Frantz et al. (2018) showed a Euclidian distance error of 6.27mm for -90° and 6.90mm for 90° during spatial alignment assessment. This is superior to the results of the Jux3DModel AR HMD system for both procedures, although their project does not reach the 2mm requirement.

Finally, the change in the spatial misalignment result between procedure 1 and procedure 2 is a point of concern. However, no study could be found in the literature that assesses the change in the spatial map vs spatial alignment. As such the results reported here could not be compared with the literature. Further assessment is required with different settings to the SpatialMapping prefab to allow for further clarification of the results.

5.5 The spatial stability of the Jux3DModel AR HMD system

The repeated movement of HoloLens was used to analyse the virtual object's stability, with the comparison between made after the introduction of user calibration.

5.5.1 The processed results

The corresponding movement of the grid board was performed to complete the measurement procedures. To assess the stability of the application to keep the virtual object anchored, the top left corner of the virtual cube was captured for all of the PA2 photos as well (see Table A.9, Appendix A.4). The Euclidean displacement between the top left corners of the virtual cubes in P_{A1} and P_{A2} photos were then calculated by subtracting the XY coordinates from each other, with the top left corner of the real-world cube being deemed as the starting point. The Euclidian distance between the top left corners of the virtual objects in P_{A1} and P_{A2} ranged from 1.315mm to 3.285mm for the trials.

The position of the virtual cube's top right corner was also captured for all of the PB2 photos (see Table A.9, Appendix A.4). For P_{B1} vs P_{B2}, the Euclidian distance error ranged from 0.592mm to 4.479mm. The relevant displacement errors are all reported in Table 5.5.

Table 5.5: Difference in position between the top left corners of the virtual cubes for P_{A1} vs P_{A2} and P_{B1} vs P_{B2} (top right corner in the picture).

Description			
PA1 vs PA2	**Euclidian distance error (mm)**	**Y-axis displacement error (mm)**	**X-axis displacement error (mm)**
P1 T1 - P_{A1} vs P_{A2}	1.315	1.154	0.630
P1 T2 - P_{A1} vs P_{A2}	2.973	-1.051	-2.781
P1 T3 - P_{A1} vs P_{A2}	1.055	0.392	-0.979
P2 T1 - P_{A1} vs P_{A2}	3.285	2.485	-2.149
P2 T2 - P_{A1} vs P_{A2}	1.317	0.401	1.255
P2 T3 - P_{A1} vs P_{A2}	1.675	0.031	-1.675
PB1 vs PB2	**Euclidian distance error (mm)**	**Y-axis displacement error (mm)**	**Z-axis displacement error (mm)**
P1 T1 - P_{B1} vs P_{B2}	2.372	2.256	-0.732
P1 T2 - P_{B1} vs P_{B2}	4.479	0.966	-4.373
P1 T3 - P_{B1} vs P_{B2}	2.131	0.762	-1.990
P 2 T1 - P_{B1} vs P_{B2}	0.592	0.404	-0.433
P 2 T2 - P_{B1} vs P_{B2}	1.612	0.559	-1.511
P 2 T3 - P_{B1} vs P_{B2}	3.126	0.463	-3.092

5.5.2 Discussion of the spatial stability results

The spatial stability of the Jux3DModel AR HMD system has not met the required 2mm point to point accuracy constraint. For both procedures, the Jux3DModel application performed better than the native HoloLens's Holograms application. To compare with a similar spatial stability test in the literature, Vassallo et al. (2017) reported a mean error of 5.73mm and a standard deviation of 0.93mm between the locations of the virtual object after walking 7m away and back to the virtual object during their project.

5.6 The FPS rendering

The Jux3DModel AR HRM system surpassed the required 30fps requirement during all trials as detailed in the capture of the FPS visualization (see Table A.9, Appendix A.4), even with the larger 3D arm virtual object (Please see https://youtu.be/_z9KRGpczbk for the MRC video captured of the user calibration of the virtual 3 D arm). However, the large registration and alignment errors have made the user calibration AR HMD system unfit for intra-surgical guidance.
unfit for intra-surgical guidance.

Chapter 6: Fiducial marker tracking for virtual object registration with an AR HMD system

The AR HMD system (JuxFiducial) was developed to assess the fiducial marker tracking approach of registering virtual objects to real-world objects.

6.1 The JuxFiducial AR HMD system

In the absence of an external optical tracker with fiducial reflective markers, the JuxFiducial AR HMD system was developed with the Vuforia SDK (version 7.0.50) in combination with Unity and the MRTK SDK. The Vuforia SDK enabled the identification of a fiducial marker (in the form as a template marker) placed in the real-world scene to identify the pose of the real-world object. The 3D arm volume and cube were imported and added as Game Objects in the Unity scene hierarchy. With the proprietary Vuforia components added, the pose of the virtual object could be specified in relation to the template marker (target image) in the Unity virtual world scene. Figure 6.1 details the location of the template marker at the base of the hand of the 3D virtual arm model. The template marker was created as a 50x50mm square target image and was added to the Vuforia Library via the online dashboard. With Vuforia, the unit scale is in meters, i.e. the value 1 = 1m. For the 50x50mm target image, a value of 0.05 was entered as the width of the target image in scene units. The required Vuforia asset database was downloaded and added to the Unity application as an asset package.

To detect the pose of the real-world object, the built-in Vuforia computer vision package processes the real-world footage to identify the features of the specified target image. The Vuforia image processing algorithms also assess the scale of the target image captured from the real-world footage. These processes are instantaneous. As soon as the target image is identified, the virtual object(s) are rendered in the FOV of the user (clinician) according to the predefined pose of the virtual objects specified in the Unity virtual world scene; at the computed scale.

Vuforia's Extended Tracking (Figure 6.1) is the counterpart of the spatial mapping process performed by the HoloLens. As such, the SpatialMapping prefab was not added during the initial setup of the Unity scene when the MRTK settings were applied.

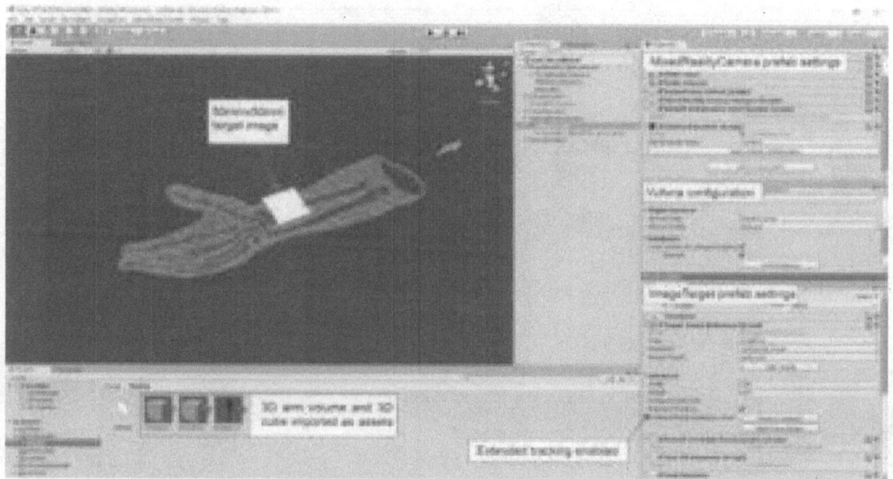

Figure 6.1: Image of the JuxFiducial Unity application with the pose of 3D arm volume (the virtual object) specified in relation to the pose of the fiducial template marker. The location of the Extended Tracking setting in Unity is illustrated.

The JuxFiducial AR HMD system specifications are represented as a process flow in Figure 6.2 (a). As shown in Figure 6.2 (b) it was feasible to use fiducial marker tracking to align the 3D virtual arm to the 3D printed hand using a fabricated target imageboard. With the extend tracking feature enabled the virtual object could be kept at the last pose recorded with the observation of the target image even after it had been removed. However, any detected movement of the target image in the real-world footage would result in the virtual object being moved. As such, the fiducial marker tracking system could possibly be used to solve for the patient moving use case, however, in the case of tissue deformation the movement of the marker could lead to inaccuracies.

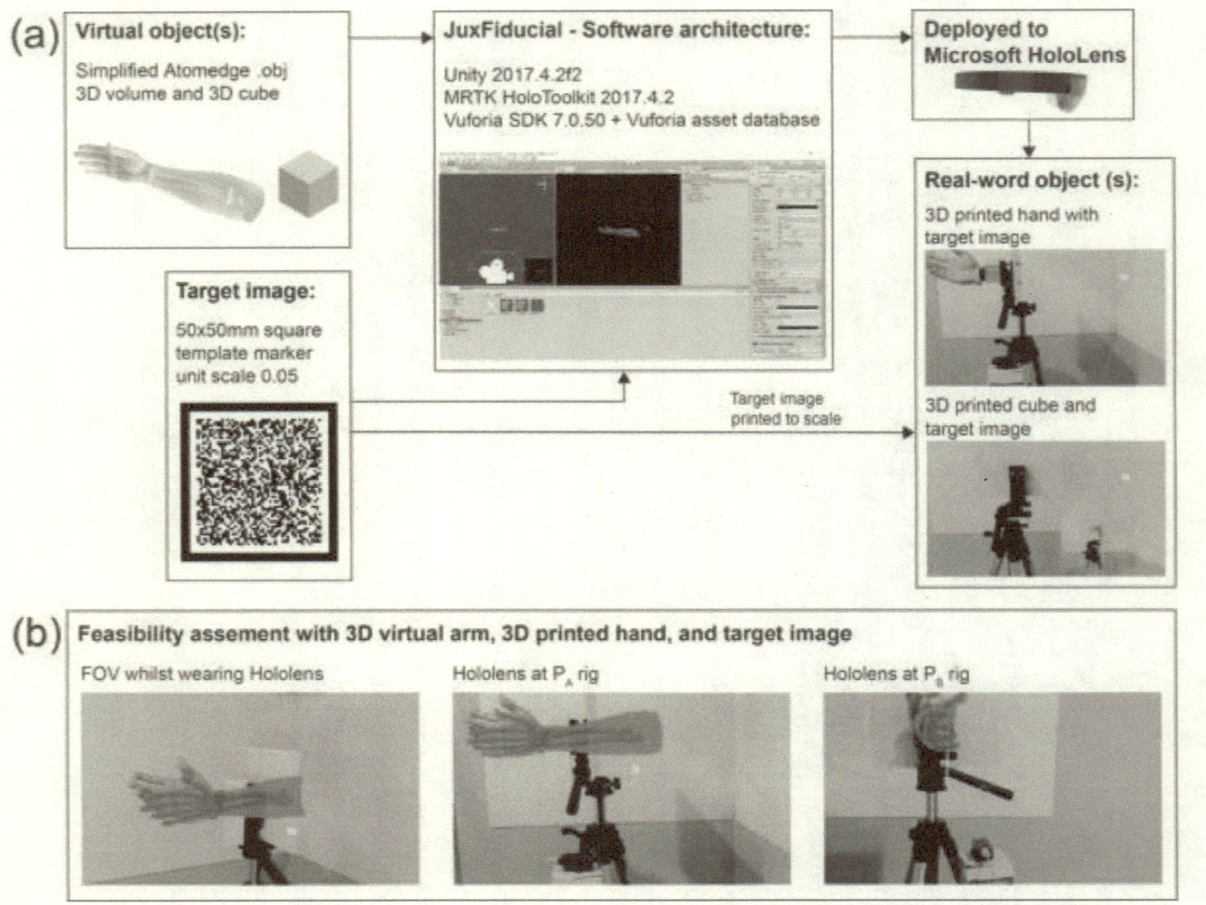

Figure 6.2: Process flow of the JuxFiducial AR HMD system to access fiducial marker tracking.

6.2 JuxFiducial AR HMD system assessment

For quantitative assessment, the virtual cube was constrained to be behind (below) the target image in the Unity scene (Figure 6.3 (a)). The combined target image and 3D cube Game Object was placed a 100cm away from the FOV origin (MixedRealityCamera prefab assembly) as shown in the Unity scene setup in Figure 6.3 (b).

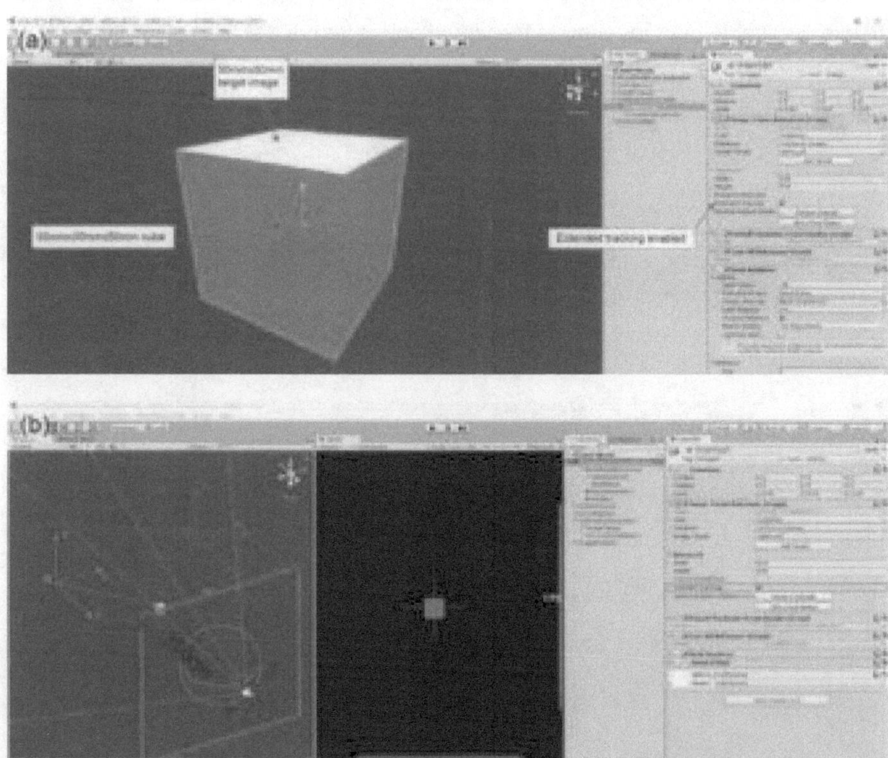

Figure 6.3: Annotations of the JuxFiducial application with the real and virtual coordinate systems depicted. (a) The 3D cube was aligned behind the target image. (b) The virtual scene was specified to match the real-world coordinates.

With the HoloLens located on the P_A rig, the JuxFiducial application was launched and MRC P_{LA} photo captured (Figure 6.4 (a)). It was expected by placing the target imageboard on the front of the real-world cube, the 50x50x50mm virtual cube would be registered to the required real-environment location in the XY-plane. However, this was not the case, as shown by the MRC P_{MC} photo (Figure 6.4 (b)); the virtual cube was not rendered into the real-world scene. The HoloLens had to be removed from the P_A rig and moved closer to P_C to detect the target image. With the HoloLens being worn by the author located between P_A and P_C, the virtual cube was rendered as required as soon as the target image was identified, and the MRC P_{FA} photo captured (Figure 6.4 (c)). There is no clear documentation on the required scale or size of the template marker, as such further analysis is required on the size of the template marker to enable the rendering of the virtual object from a distance of a 100cm.

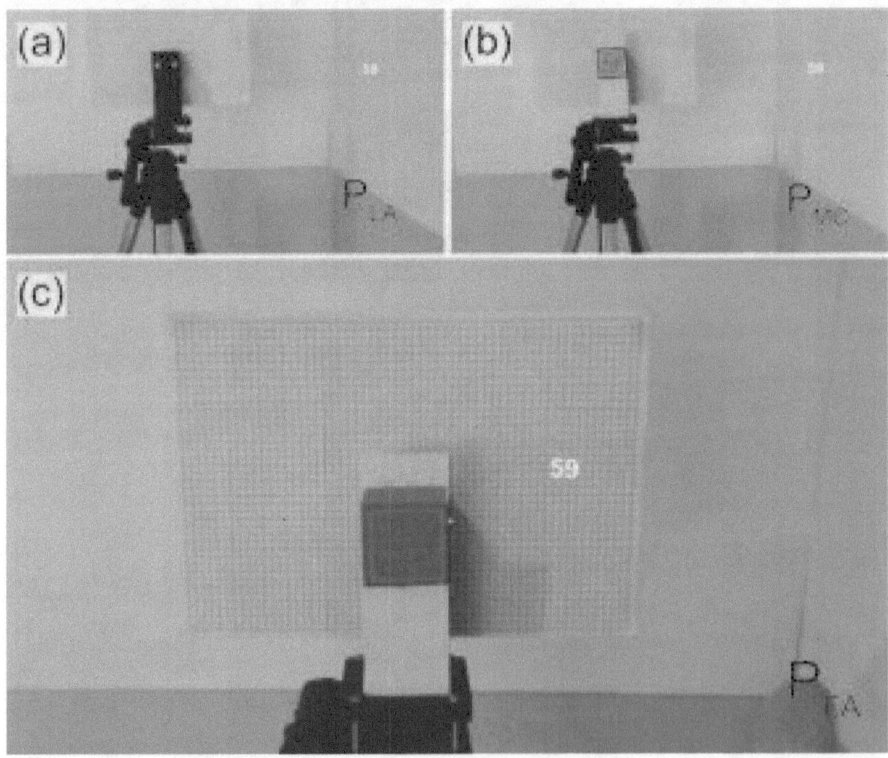

Figure 6.4: The launch of the JuxFiducial application. (a)The MRC P_{LA} photo captured directly after the launch of the application. (b) The target image placed at P_C for MRC photo P_{MC} (c) The HoloLens had to be removed from the P_A rig and brought closer to detect the target image to allow for the rendering of the virtual cube (MRC P_{FA} photo).

The target imageboard was fabricated by combining a 1:1 scale printing of the custom target image and a 150x50x4mm section of hardboard as shown below (Figure 6.5) and the updated test rig schematic is depicted in Figure 6.6.

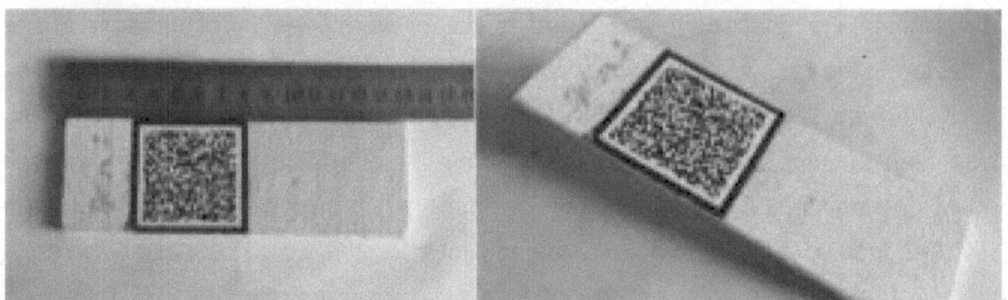

Figure 6.5: Target imageboard: 1:1 scale printing of the custom target image on a 150x50x4mm piece of hardboard.

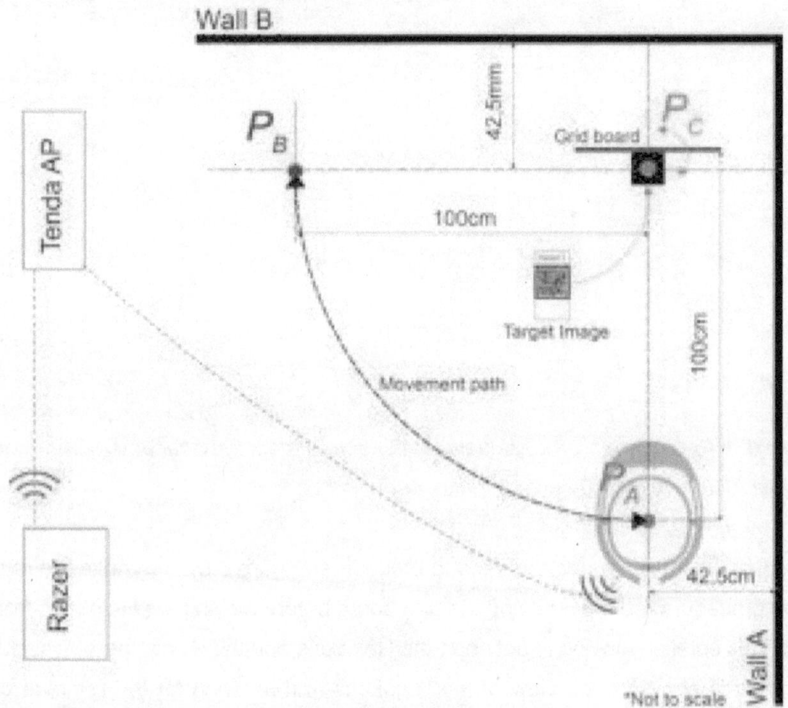

Figure 6.6: Test area schematic detailing the location of the components during the JuxFiducial AR HMD system experiment.

After capturing the P_{FA} photo, the HoloLens was placed back at the P_A rig and the MRC P_{A1} photo was captured. With the target imageboard in place, the registration between the real and virtual cube could not be measured, as the distinction between the virtual and real-world cube could not be processed in the P_{A1} photo. Consequently, the target image had to be removed and as stated, any movement of the target image detected in the real-world footage would result in the virtual object being moved. As such, to remove the target image, for the first procedure (Figure 6.7) the HoloLens was moved counter-clockwise through 90° from P_A to P_B before the template marker could be removed. An argument can be made that through use of occlusion the template marker could have been removed. However, this would not have adhered to the constant spatial map specification of the first procedure requirements detailed in chapter 4 section 9.2.

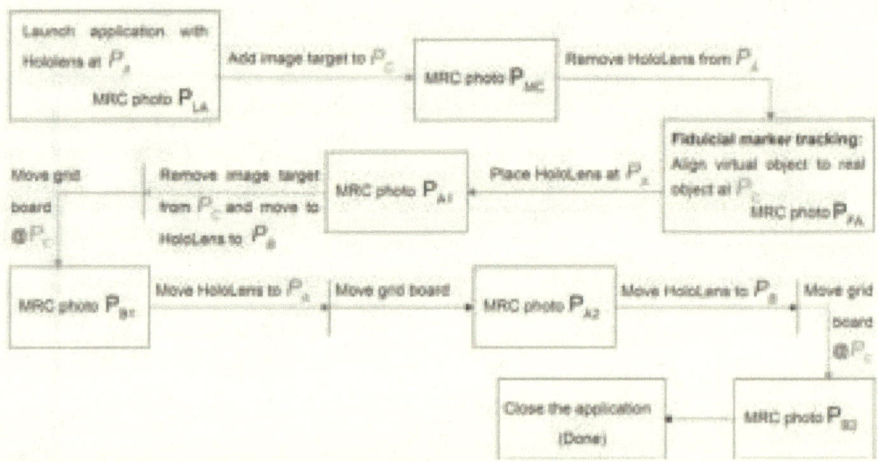

Figure 6.7: Procedure 1 process flow to simulate a stable spatial environment during the JuxFiducial AR HMD system trials.

Occlusion was used during the second procedure (Figure 6.8) to remove the marker, as the procedure required moving the grid board before moving the HoloLens from P_A to P_B. This entailed moving in between the HoloLens and the P_A rig, thereby occluding the target image from the view of the HoloLens and allowing for the removal of the target imageboard and the rotation of the grid board.

The process of moving of the HoloLens closer to the P_C rig to allow the rendering of the virtual cube did not conform to the previously specified procedure flows, as such, the MRC P_{LB} photo was not captured for either procedure. With the Extended Tracking function feature enabled the virtual object was kept at the last pose recorded with the observation of the target image during both procedures.

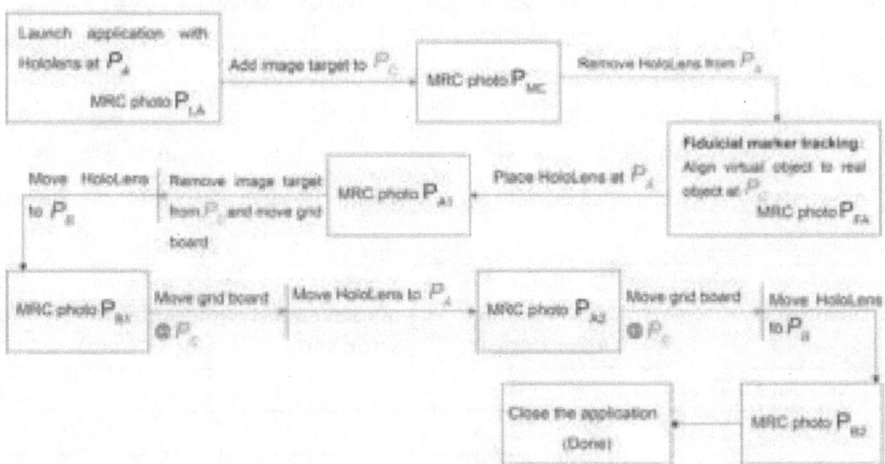

Figure 6.8: Procedure 2 process flow to simulate a change in the environment that the captured virtual spatial map needs to adapt for during the JuxFiducial AR HMD system trials.

6.3 Registration accuracy at P_A

Without the capture of the MRC photo at the launch of the JuxFiducial AR HMD system, the virtual to real-world calibration could not be measured, rather as discussed, the MRC P_{A2} photo had to be used to determine the accuracy of the fiducial protocol registration. To quantitatively calculate the registration accuracy the Euclidean displacement between the top left corners of the real and virtual cube was measured in the corresponding procedure's XY plane P_{A2} photos. The Euclidean displacement error between the top left corners of the real and virtual cube ranged from 0mm for procedure 1 - trial 1 (Figure 6.9 (a)) to a maximum identified error of 3.053mm for procedure 2 - trial 1 (Figure 6.9 (b)). All the relevant point assessment errors identified are reported in Table 6.1.

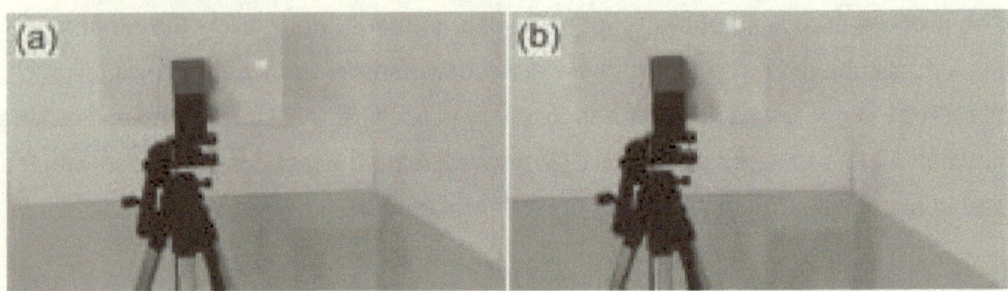

Figure 6.9: Registration errors identified during the assessment of the JuxFiducial application. (a) P_{A2} of procedure 1 trial 2. (b) P_{A2} of procedure 2 trial 1; the arrow shows the error's vector direction.

Table 6.1: Difference in position between the top left corners of the real cube and the virtual cube at P_{A1}.

Description	Euclidian displacement error (mm)	Y-axis displacement error (mm)	X-axis displacement error (mm)
Procedure 1 Trial 1	0	0	0
Procedure 1 Trial 2	0	0	0
Procedure 1 Trial 3	1.214	-0.899	-0.819
Procedure 2 Trial 1	3.053	-1.672	2.553
Procedure 2 Trial 2	0	0	0
Procedure 2 Trial 3	3.018	-1.755	-2.387

6.3.1 Discussion of accuracy results

Specifying the displacement between the virtual camera and the target image had no influence on the final result as Vuforia did not take the measurement into account when placing the virtual object in the FOV. As shown by procedure 1 trial 2, if the fiducial marker (target image) is correctly aligned to the real-world object, the JuxFiducial application can register the virtual object to the real-world object within the 2mm requirement. Frantz et al. (2018) noted registration errors during the assessment of their cylindrical tarmac image marker tracking application as smaller than 5mm for all of their trials. With the largest point error measurement of 3.05mm in the case of correct point target alignment the JuxFiducial AR HMD system performed on par with the Frantz study. However, with fiducial marking care needs to be taken when aligning the target image, as any deviation in an accurate calibration leads to registration errors as shown in the result of procedure 1 trial 3, procedure 2 trial 1 and 3.

6.4 Spatial alignment at P_B

To assess the spatial alignment of the JuxFiducial AR HMD system the HoloLens was moved counter-clockwise through 90° from P_A to P_B and placed on the P_B rig to capture the MRC P_{B1} photo (Figure 6.10). For procedure 1 the grid board and removal of the fiducial marker was rotated after this movement, whilst for procedure 2 the grid board rotation and the removal of the fiducial marker preceded the movement of the HoloLens through occluding the view of the target image from the HoloLens as stated above. To qualitatively calculate the spatial alignment accuracy, the Euclidean displacement between the top left corners of the real and virtual cube identified in the XY plane was measured in the YZ plane using the P_{B1} photo (i.e. the right corners in the P_{B1} photo). The image target board had a 4mm thickness, as such in theory the results should have shown a spatial alignment error of 4mm between the real and virtual cube on the Z-axis. However, the Euclidean displacement between the top corners of the real and virtual cubes all showed a negative Z-axis error, with the largest being -4.132mm for procedure 2 - trial 1 (see Figure 6.10 (a)). For Procedure 2 trial 3 the top right corners had an indistinguishable error, however, as shown Figure 6.10 (b) all three of the other corners were misaligned, with the top left corners in the P_{B1} photo resulting in a Euclidian distance error of 4,48mm. All the spatial alignment errors identified are reported in Table 6.2.

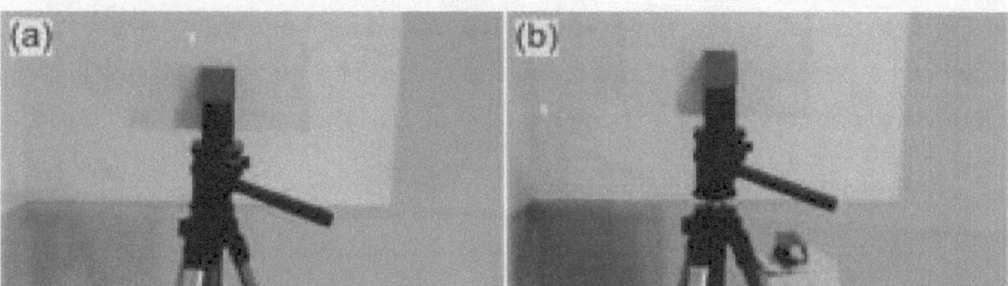

Figure 6.10: Spatial alignment errors identified in the MRC P_{B1} photos. (a) P_{B1} of procedure 1 trial 2. (b) P_{B1} of procedure 2 trial 1.

Table 6.2: Difference in position between the top left corners of the real cube and the virtual cube at P_{B1} (the top right corner in the YZ plane pictures).

Description	Euclidian distance error (mm)	Y-axis displacement error (mm)	Z-axis displacement error (mm)
Procedure 1 Trial 1	2.982	-1.659	-2.488
Procedure 1 Trial 2	3.558	-0.901	-3.446
Procedure 1 Trial 3	2.706	-0.898	-2.559
Procedure 2 Trial 1	4.225	-0.899	-4.132
Procedure 2 Trial 2	1.167	-0.824	-0.833
Procedure 2 Trial 3	0	0	0

6.4.1 Discussion of the spatial alignment results

As specified the virtual object was to be rendered with no spacing behind the target image. For JuxFiducial, the Euclidian distance error identified in the spatial alignment could be attributed to an inherent spatial drift error in the Extended Tracking function or a possible detection of the target image having been moved. However, the error is less than the Spatial Mapping error for the MRTK SDK. During both procedures, the JuxFiducial AR HMS system failed to meet the spatial alignment point to point error < 2mm requirement for except two trials, and therefore the JuxFiducial AR HMD system is unfit for intra-surgical guidance at this point in time.

Frantz et al. (2018) noted an error of 0.83mm at -90°, 1.24mm at 0°, and 3.42mm at 90° for spatial alignment. It should be noted that the target image had not been removed before or during the user movement around the virtual and real-world objects in the Franz et al. experimental setup. The JuxFiducial AR HMD system spatial alignment experiments would need to be repeated with the target image kept in place for a one-to-one comparison with the Frantz et al. (2018) study.

6.5 The spatial stability of the JuxFiducial AR HMD system

The fact that the target image occluded the real-world object in the P_{A1} photo did not deter from measuring the spatial stability of the virtual object in the XY plane. To access the stability of the JuxFiducial AR HMD system to keep the virtual object anchored in the real-world environment, the visible real-world objects in the P_{A1} and

P_{A2} photos were aligned and the Euclidean distance between the top left corners of the virtual cubes identified in the XY plane were measured for all of the trial (Figure 6.11). The real-world objects in the P_{B1} and P_{B2} photos were calculated by subtracting the vector values after measuring the displacement errors in the PB2 photos (please see Table A.10, Appendix A.4 for the P_{B2} measurements).

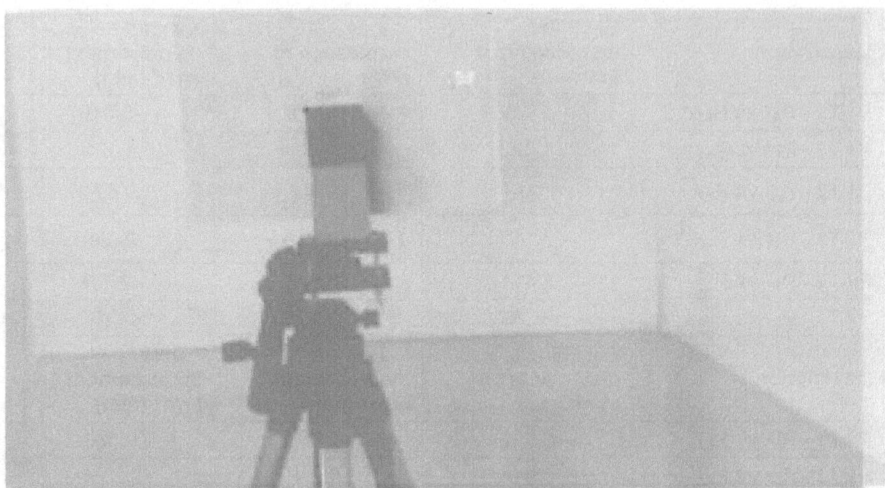

Figure 6.11: Comparison of the location of the virtual objects to assess spatial stability at P_A for Procedure 1 Trial 3. To assess the stability the real-world objects were aligned after the top left corners were marked and the displacement between the centre of the two marks was measured.

Stability assessment showed that Euclidean distance between the top left corners of the virtual objects in P_{A1} vs P_{A2} ranged from 1.494mm to 2.411mm with no specific pattern in the direction of the drift. For P_{B1} vs P_{B2}, the stability errors ranged from 0.732mm to 2.367mm. All relevant errors have been reported in Table 6.3 on the following page.

6.5.1 Discussion of the spatial stability results

The JuxFiducial AR HMD system performed better in spatial stability than the Jux3DModel AR HMD system, however for 4 out of the 12 trials the spatial stability point to point error requirement of below the 2mm was not met. Currently, there are no studies identified, in the medical realm, that asses the stability of virtual objects registered through marker tracking to the real-world object during multiple movements of the user (clinician) wearing an AR HMD.

Table 6.3: Difference in position between the top left corners of the virtual cubes for P_{A1} vs P_{A2} and P_{B1} vs P_{B2} (top right corner in the picture).

Description	Euclidian distance error (mm)	Y-axis displacement error (mm)	X-axis displacement error (mm)
P1 T1 - P_{A1} vs P_{A2}	1.781	-1.778	-0.016
P1 T2 - P_{A1} vs P_{A2}	1.822	1.460	1.100
P1 T3 - P_{A1} vs P_{A2}	1.494	1.347	0.626
P2 T1 - P_{A1} vs P_{A2}	2.140	-0.734	2.008
P2 T2 - P_{A1} vs P_{A2}	2.411	-0.925	-2.224
P2 T3 - P_{A1} vs P_{A2}	2.289	-2.107	0.017
Description	**Euclidian distance error (mm)**	**Y-axis displacement error (mm)**	**Z-axis displacement error (mm)**
P1 T1 - P_{B1} vs P_{B2}	0.732	0.727	0.086
P1 T2 - P_{B1} vs P_{B2}	0.914	-0.897	0.174
P1 T3 - P_{B1} vs P_{B2}	0.829	-0.822	0.107
P 2 T1 - P_{B1} vs P_{B2}	1.799	-0.794	1.614
P 2 T2 - P_{B1} vs P_{B2}	0.811	-0.020	-0.810
P 2 T3 - P_{B1} vs P_{B2}	2.367	-1.685	-1.662

6.6 FPS Discussion of results

The JuxFiducial AR HMD system met the 30 or more fps requirement during all trials (see Table A.10). The large spatial alignment error nevertheless deems the system unfit for intra-surgical guidance. If the spatial alignment and stability capabilities are improved the JuxFiducial AR HMD system could possibly be used for AR registration during intra-surgical guidance as both the initial alignment, spatial alignment and the spatial stability results showed errors below the 2mm requirement. However, more in-depth system performance measurements, accuracy assessments, and adaptability to real-world scenario tests are required to fully detail the feasibility of the JuxFiducial AR HMD system for intra-surgical guidance.

Chapter 7: Markerless tracking for virtual object registration with an AR HMD system

The final AR HMD system developed, JuxL_Combo, is a markerless tracking system which combines the Microsoft HoloLens with Leap Motion's hand-tracking sensor, the Leap Motion Controller (LMC). The 3D printed hand was used as the real-world hand to be tracked via the LMC.

7.1 The JuxL_Combo AR HMD system

As discussed in chapter 4 section 4.3 the LMC is a small rectangular box measuring 75×25×6.2mm and makes use of infrared light-emitting diodes and monochromatic infra-red cameras to enable tracking of the lower arm. To process the pose data of the 3D printed hand the LMC needs to be connected to a separate processing device via Universal Serial Bus (USB) configured with the Leap Motion Orion SDK. Although the HoloLens has a USB mini port it does not support external peripherals. Consequently, a Razer Blade Stealth Laptop (2018) was configured with the Orion SDK for Windows. Part of the Orion SDK is Leap Motion's proprietary setup software that handles the processing of the pose data of the tracked real-world object. Also, the Leap Motion Core Assets 4.4.0 SDK for Unity that enabled the porting of the processed pose data to the JuxL_Combo Unity built application running on the Razer Laptop. Making use of the Leap Motion Core prefabs, the real-world pose could be dynamically visualized in the JuxL_Combo Unity virtual scene.

The Razer and the HoloLens were wirelessly connected via a local area network (LAN) using a Tenda Wi-Fi Router. The Holographic Remoting Player (HRP) application enabled the streaming of the real environment footage and pose data from the HoloLens to the JuxL_Combo Unity application. To create the AR visualization, the JuxL_Combo Unity application combined the FOV footage with the dynamic Capsule Hand visualization. The combined computer graphic was then rendered back to the HoloLens via the HRP application.

The HoloLens's MRC video capture feature enabled the capturing of the AR experience as shown in Figure 7.1 detailing the process flow of the JuxL_Combo AR HMD system on the following page. To align the virtual Capsule Hand with the 3D printed hand in the FOV, the correct transformation matrix is required. Unfortunately, the Orion SDK does not support automated alignment. User calibration or fiducial marker tracking provide alternatives to the automated alignment. The assessment of the Jux3D_Model and the JuxFiducial AR HMD systems showed that the performance of Vuforia's Extended tracking system in maintaining the pose of the virtual object in spatial alignment is superior to MRTK's SpatialMapping prefab at default settings. For the Vuforia engine to detect the target image, it takes control over the MixedRealityCamera module and disables the possibility of streaming to and from the HoloLens via the HRP application in Unity. Therefore, to align the virtual object to the real-world object, user calibration had to be used similar to the Jux3DModel AR HMD system. The notable prefabs that were used in the development of the JuxL_Combo Unity application are detailed in Table 7.1 below.

Table 7.1: Notable Leap Motion Core prefabs used in combination with the MRTK

Leap Motion Core prefab	**Description**
LeapHandController	Queries the Leap Motion service for tracking data and uses it to place hands in the scene. The tracking data from the service is transformed relative to the prefab's position and orientation in the scene. The scripts in the controller manage the hand objects that represent the physical hands detected by the Leap Motion device.
RigidRoundHand	Includes a rigid body and collider composition of for the arm, palm and all of the digits so to animate the graphic visualization
Capsule Hand	Dynamic graphic visualization to be combined with RigidroundHand

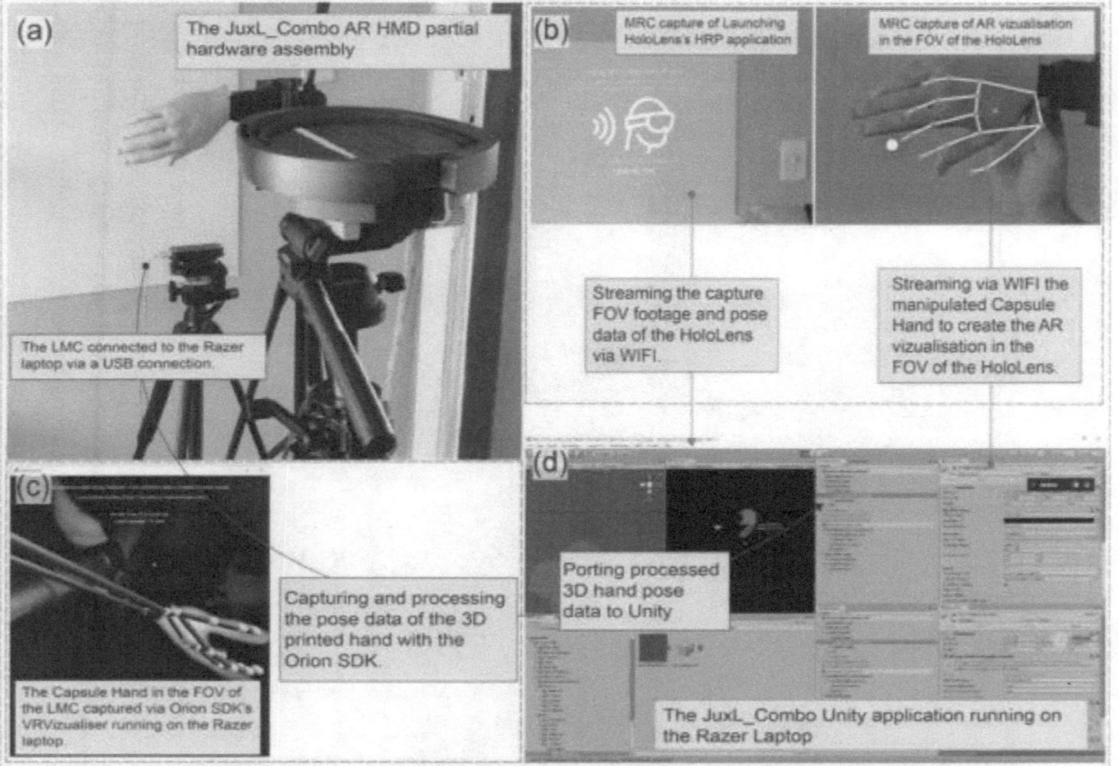

Figure 7.1: Hardware and software assembly of the JuxL_Combo AR HMD system to evaluate markerless tracking. (a) The HoloLens, the LMC, 3D printed hand and tripod rigs. (b) MRC captures of the HoloLens's FOV. (c) The Capsule Hand in the FOV of the LMC captured via Orion SDK's VRVizualiser running on the Razer laptop. (d) The JuxL_Combo Unity application running on the Razer laptop.

By running the Unity application on the Razer instead of deploying it to the HoloLens, it was possible to align the virtual and real objects through changing the transform values of the LeapHandController (renamed Leap Motion Controller in the Unity scene) prefab in the Unity scene (see Figure 7.2).

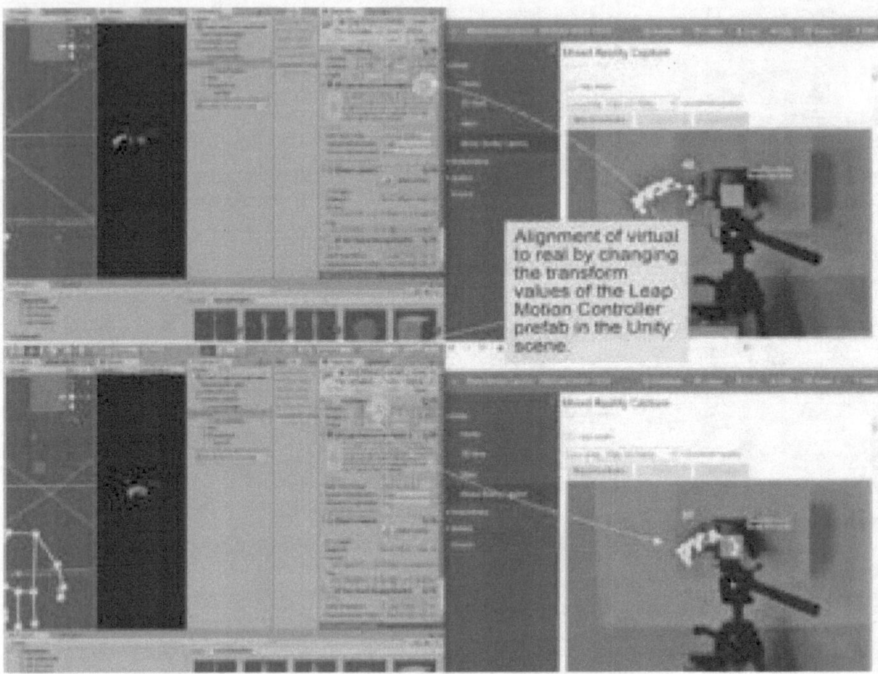

Figure 7.2: Aligning the virtual Capsule Hand visualization with the 3D printed hand in the MRC video streamed via HoloLens's device portal by changing the transform values of the LeapHandController prefab in the Unity scene.

By changing the transform values, only the pose alignment of the virtual hand was influenced and not the markerless tracking of the hand. In other words, when the hand was rotated, the LeapHandController's transform values did not change. This allowed for calibration of the LMC's FOV Cartesian coordinate transformation values with regard to the FOV of the HoloLens; represented by the MixedRealityCamera prefab in the virtual scene. As such, using the LMC to simulate markerless tracking in combination with the HoloLens was deemed feasible.

7.2 JuxL_Combo AR HMD system calibration

The rig at P_C was updated to include a 50x50x50mm cube, the 3D printed hand, a grid board and the LMC. With markerless tracking of the 3D printed hand enabled, it was theorised that the AR view through the HoloLens would be a dynamic juxtaposed view of the Orion SDK's Capsule Hand in real-time. The updated test rig schematic is represented in Figure 7.3.

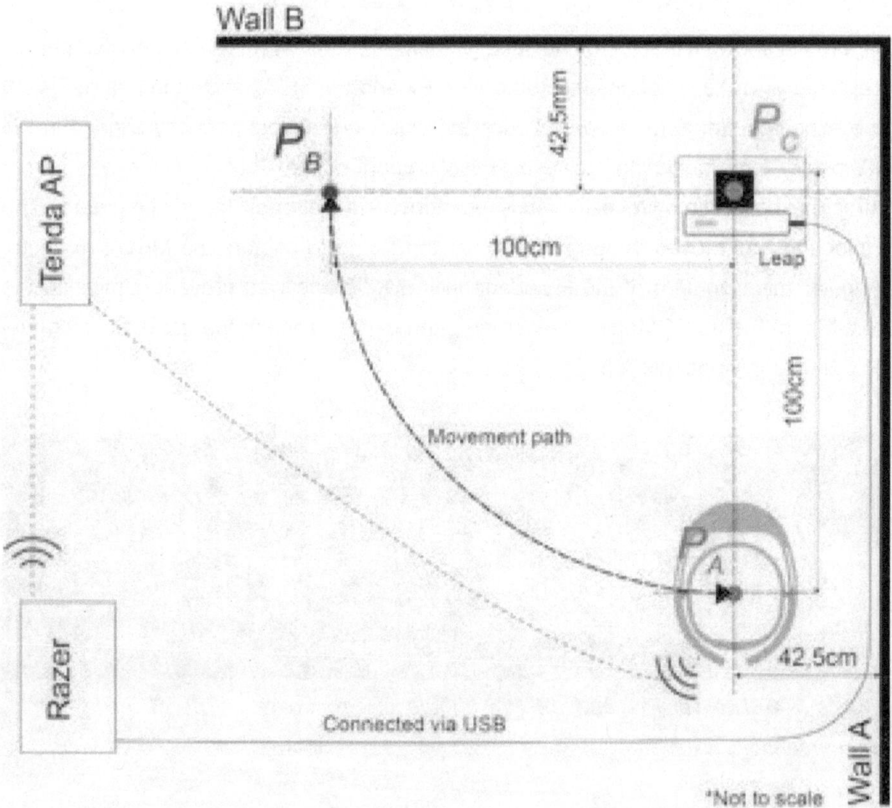

Figure 7.3: Layout of the test rig to assess the JuxL_Combo AR HMD system.

The virtual scene content (FPS prefab, 3D cube and 3D arm model) of JuxL_Combo was all set to be rendered a 100cm away from the MixedRealityCameraParent prefab. The virtual cube was to be rendered 25mm to the left of the real cube as shown in on the X-axis. To calibrate the launch location of the Capsule Hand, the HoloLens was placed on the P_A rig in the calibrated real-world environment. A combination of the JuxL_Combo Unity application and the MRC dashboard was used to enable user calibration of the Capsule Hand visualisation and the 3D printed hand alignment in the XY plane. This process was only completed once, and the transform values of the LeapHandController prefab were kept constant during all trials.

7.3 JuxL_combo AR HMD system assessment

Figure 7.4 shows a trial run of the JuxL_Combo AR HMD system with the MRC photos captured with the HoloLens located on the P_A and P_B rig. As shown in Figure 7.4 (a) the expected virtual to real-world cube settings were almost perfectly aligned in the XY-plane upon launching, however, misalignment of the Capsule Hand was visible after the calibration process discussed above had already been completed. The HoloLens was moved through 90° CW to the P_B rig to capture the MRC P_{LB} photo. Angular misalignment of the HoloLens in the XZ-plane was present, similar to the result from the Jux3DModel assessment, and can be seen in the corresponding trial P_{LB} photos in Appendix A.3.

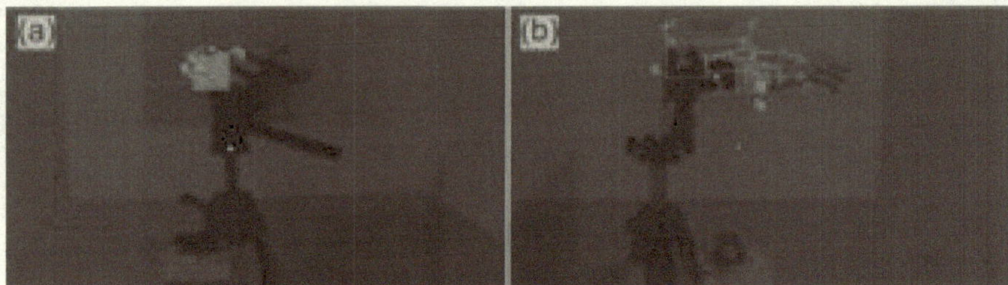

Figure 7.4: The (a) P_{LA} and (b) P_{LB} photos of Procedure 1 Trial 3 JuxL_Combo experiments.

As such, it was decided to eliminate the misalignment errors captured in the P_{LA} and P_{LB} photos with user calibration (Air tap and hold) to align the virtual and real-world objects before placing the HoloLens back on the P_A rig, these steps were completed during would be completed for all of the procedure trials.

To determine the scale measurement via the gird board the entire head of the tripod rig had to be rotated. In other words, the tripods rotating head mount was rotated around the central axis of the tripod, instead of just removing and rotating the 3D cube and grid board combination at P_C. The tripod's head mount had a 360° protractor engraved. The head was rotated from the 180° mark to the 270° mark as shown in Figure 7.5 on the next page.

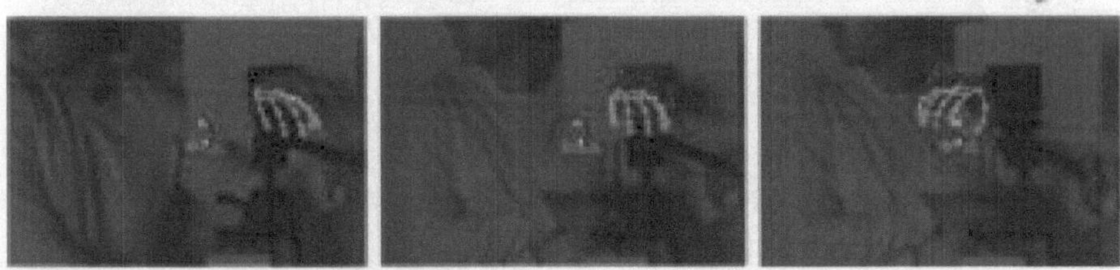

Figure 7.5: The 3d printed hand, cube, and grid board had to be rotated through 90 degrees around the central axis of the tripod using the tripods rotating head mount.

7.3.1 Procedure 1 – Constant spatial environment during movement followed with patient movement

With rotating the grid board after moving the HoloLens from P_A to P_B, the assessment procedures discussed in chapter 4 section 9 needs to be updated due to the fact that the hand also moves when the grid board is rotated to capture the registration accuracy. Procedure 1 is detailed as a process flow in Figure 7.6. To test for conforming results, three trials of the procedure were completed.

During the first trial for procedure 1, the LMC had lost the hand tracking whilst moving from P_{B1} to P_{A2}. With trial 2, there was a delay in streaming the visualization from the Razer to the HoloLens as well as the 3D printed hand tracking was lost whilst moving the rig from P_{A2} to P_{B2}. Trial 3 was the only successful experiment.

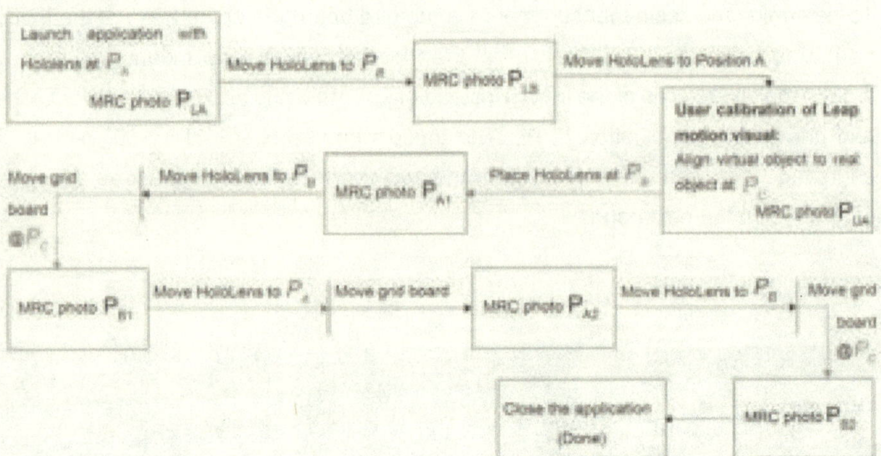

Figure 7.6: Procedure 1 process flow to simulate a stable spatial environment during the JuxL_Combo AR HMD system trials.

The loss of the Capsule Hand visual can be attributed to the LMC not being able to track the 3D printed hand due to inefficient IR light reflection from the surface of the 3D printed hand (Figure 7.7).

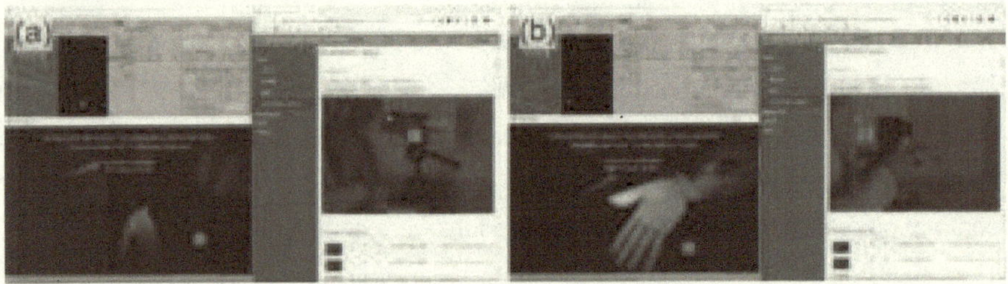

Figure 7.7: Leap Motion markerless tracking loss. (a) Loss of tracking with HoloLens at PA. (b) Loss of tracking wit HoloLens at PB.

The 3D printed hand had been spray-painted a different colour as there was little to no light reflection from the original black filament. Although the change in colour resulted in greater stability of reflection, the loss of markerless tracking happened as seen during trial 1 and 2 of procedure 1. For non-simulated environments, this could lead to irregularities when persons with different skin tone need to make use of the

LMC rig setup and has been noted as a point of concern for future work. Evaluation of the measured results led to selecting trial 3 for procedure 1 as this was the only successfully completed trial.

7.3.2 Procedure 2 – Change in the spatial environment before moving around the real-world object

Procedure 2 mirrors the simulation procedure discussed in chapter 6 section 4.2. Even though the hand rotates with the grid board, this would be deemed as part of a change in the spatial environment. Procedure 2 is represented in Figure 7.8 as a process flow to detail the sequence of MRC photos captured.

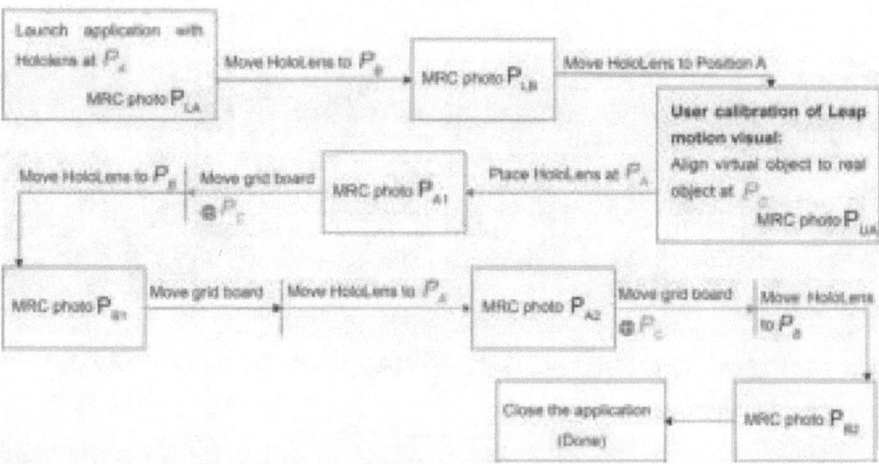

Figure 7.8: Procedure 2's process flow to simulate a change in the spatial environment during the JuxL_Combo AR HMD system trials.

For Procedure 2 trial 1, the Capsule Hand visual was lost whilst moving from P_{B1} to P_{A2}. For trial 2, there was a delay in the streaming between the HoloLens and the Razer, which resulted in the loss of the AR visual during the capture of P_{LA}, P_{LB} and P_{UA}. Once again, trial 3 was the only completely successful trial.

7.4 Registration accuracy after user calibration registration of the markerless tracking system P_A

The MRC function was used to capture the P_{A1} photo. As the qualitative experiment virtual and real object had changed from the cube to the virtual Capsule Hand and 3D printed hand, the Euclidean distance between the centre point of the Capsule Hand thumb's distal end to the perceived centre point of the distal end of the 3D printed thumb was measured in the XY plane using the P_{A1} photo. The Euclidian distance between the centres of the distal end of the 3D printed thumb and virtual Capsule thumb visualizations was 35.98mm for procedure 1 - trial 3, and 38.26mm for procedure 2 - trial 3 (Figure 7.9). The relevant displacements are reported in Table 7.2.

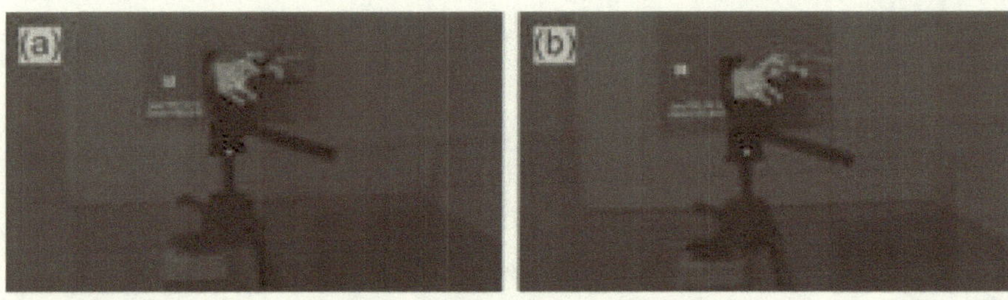

Figure 7.9: Assessment of registration errors identified between Capsule Hand visualization and 3D printed hand in the P_{A1} MRC photos. (a) P_{A1} of procedure 1 trial 3. (b) P_{A1} of procedure 2 trial 3.

Table 7.2: Difference in position between the centres of the real and virtual thumb at P_{A1}.

Description	Euclidian distance error (mm)	Y-axis displacement error (mm)	X-axis displacement error (mm)	FPS
Procedure 1 Trial 3	35.98	-1.69	-35.93	32
Procedure 2 Trial 1	38.26	6.15	-37.75	38

7.4.1 Discussion of results

The registration alignment error found in P_{A1} between the virtual Capsule thumb visual and the distal end of the 3D printed thumb can be attributed to an inherent tracking error of in either the Capsule Hand visualisation or the LMC. The tracking visualisation does not follow the contour of the thumb, as shown in Figure 7.10 (a) for the 3D printed hand, or a real hand (Figure 7.10 (b)).

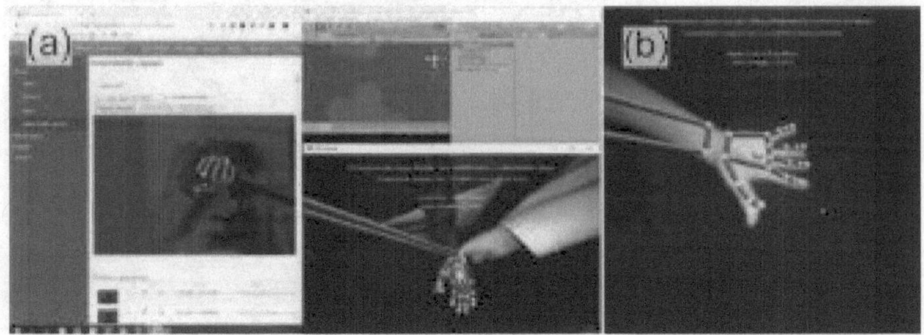

Figure 7.10: Error in the thumb contour identified in the Capsule Hand visualization. (a) Error for the 3D printed hand. (b) Error for a human hand.

7.5 Spatial alignment accuracy at P_B

To qualitatively calculate the spatial alignment accuracy, the Euclidean distance between the centre point of the Capsule Hand thumb visualisation to the perceived centre point of the distal end of the 3D printed thumb was measured in the YZ plane in the P_{B1} photo. The Euclidean distance between the centre point of the Capsule Hand thumb visualisation and the perceived centre point of the distal end of the 3D printed thumb in P_{B1} was 170.05mm for procedure 1 - trial 3, detailed in the PB1 marker MRC capture in Figure 7.11. For procedure 2 - trial 3, the P_{B2} photo was used since the starting pose of the hand could only be captured at the end of the trial. In Figure 7.12 the P_{B2} marked photo, the spatial alignment error was 228.38mm. Both figures detail the spatial drift error between the simulated movement. The relevant errors are reported in Table 7.3.

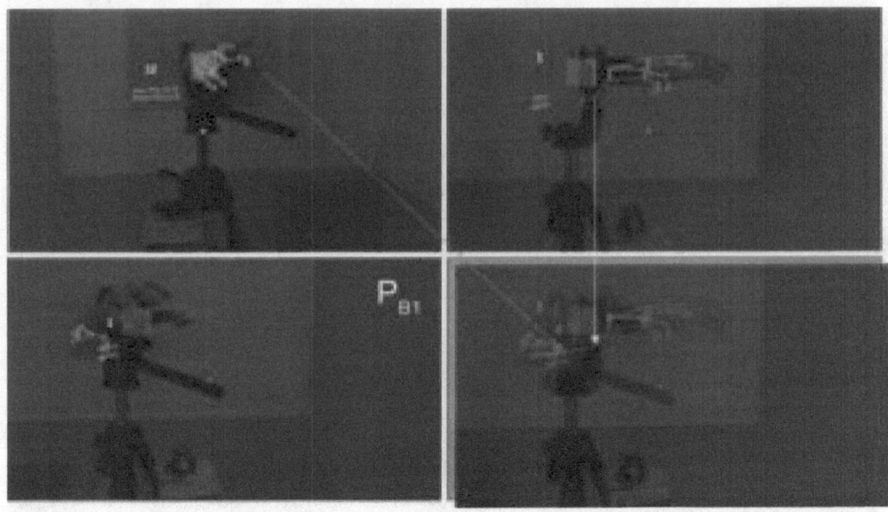

Figure 7.11: Spatial alignment error identified in the P_{B1} MRC photo for procedure 1 trial 3.

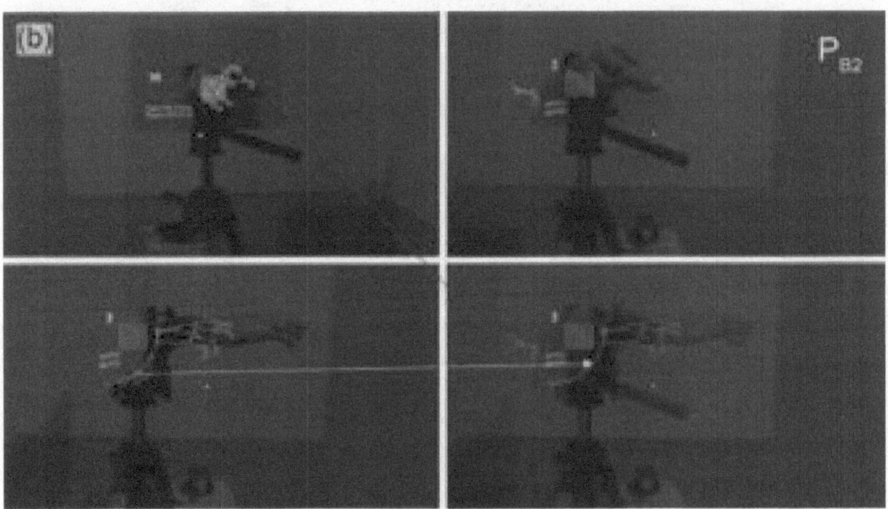

Figure 7.12: The spatial alignment errors identified in the P_{B2} MRC photo for procedure 2 trial 3.

Table 7.3: Difference in position between the top left corners of the real cube and the virtual cube at P_{B1} (the top right corner in the YZ plane pictures).

Description	Euclidian distance error (mm)	Y-axis displacement error (mm)	Z-axis displacement error (mm)	FPS
Procedure 1 Trial 3	170.05	-61.27	-158.65	36
Procedure 2 Trial 3	228.38	-32.08	-226.10	37

7.5.1 Discussion of results

The registration error in P_{A1} combined with the inherent spatial drift error of the MRTK spatial map function resulted in the spatial misalignment in P_{B2} as depicted in Figure 7.11 and Figure 7.12. The LMC did not relocate the visualization and further research is required to set up the sensor as an outside-in optical tracking system (see section 4.5.1).

7.6 Spatial stability

To assess the spatial stability of the JuxL_Combo application the HoloLens was moved back to P_A and once again to P_B. For procedure 1, the grid board was rotated after this movement whilst for procedure 2, the grid board rotation preceded the movement of the HoloLens. The spatial stability results are detailed in the comparison of the P_{A1} vs P_{A2} and the P_{B1} vs P_{B2} assessments. To assess the stability of the application to keep the virtual object anchored in the spatial environment, the Euclidean distance between the centre point of the corresponding Capsule Hand thumb visualisations were measured.

The Euclidian distance between the centres of the virtual Capsule Hand thumbs in P_{A1} and P_{A2} was 17.40mm for procedure 1 - trial 3, and 17.35mm for procedure 2 - trial 3 (Figure 7.13 (a) and (b)). For P_{B1} vs P_{B2}, the Euclidian distance error was 13.36 mm for procedure 1 trial 3, and 14.10mm for procedure 2 trial 3 (Figure 7.13 (c) and (d)). The relevant displacement errors are reported in Table 7.4.

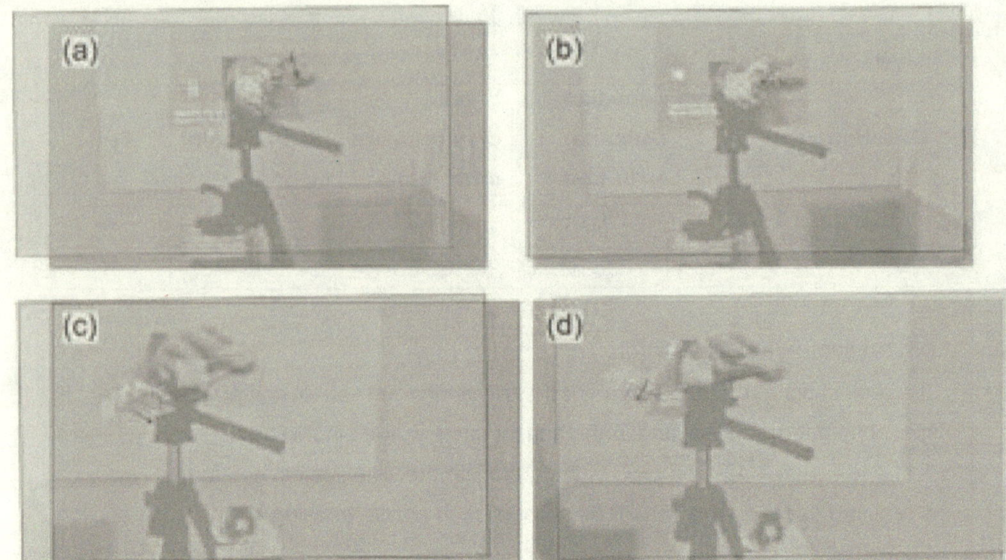

Figure 7.13: Change in the pose of virtual Capsule Hands to assess spatial stability. (a) P_{A1} vs P_{A2} of procedure 1 trial 3. (b) P_{A1} vs P_{A2} of procedure 2 trial 3. (c) P_{B1} vs P_{B2} of procedure 1 trial 3. (d) P_{B1} vs P_{B2} of procedure 2 trial 3.

Table 7.4: Difference in position between the top left corners of the virtual cubes for P_{A1} vs P_{A2} and P_{B1} vs P_{B2} (top right corner in the picture).

Description	Euclidian distance error (mm)	Y-axis displacement error (mm)	X-axis displacement error (mm)	FPS for P_{A2}
P1 T3 - P_{A1} vs P_{A2}	17.40	-16.94	-2.91	34
P2 T3 - P_{A1} vs P_{A2}	17.35	-12.67	-11.99	36
			Z-axis (mm)	**FPS P_{B2}**
P 1 T3 - P_{B1} vs P_{B2}	13.36	-6.03	11.86	34
P2 T3 - P_{B1} vs P_{B2}	14.10	-12.83	-5.83	Unavailable

7.6.1 Discussion of results

The JuxL_Combo AR HMD system had the worst performance for spatial stability of the three AR HMD systems. However, the increase in error could be attributed to an inherent test rig fault, as the P_C rig had to be manually rotated as depicted in Figure 7.5 The trials should be repeated on a more secure rig that can assure the absolute alignment of the real-world object during rotation.

7.7 The FPS rendering

The JuxL_Combo HMD system met the minimum 30fps requirement (please see Table A.7 and A.9, Appendix A.3), but due to the inaccuracies in registration and alignment, it is also not a viable solution for intra-surgical guidance.

Chapter 8: Discussion and Conclusion

This project explored the use of computer-mediated reality technology, particularly the reconstruction and visualization of 3D patient-specific bone models for intra-surgical guidance with a commercially available AR HMD system, the Microsoft HoloLens. Three AR HMD systems were developed to explore the capabilities of the HoloLens as an AR HMD medical system. Each of the applications implemented a different registration technique to localize the virtual object in the real-world coordinate system. The registration techniques explored included user calibration, fiducial marker tracking, and markerless tracking. Assessing the registration techniques required the development of the aforementioned AR HMD systems, each requiring different software and hardware assemblies.

All three of the AR HMD system applications were developed in Unity. For user calibration with anatomical landmarks, the MRTK SDK was added to the Unity build and manipulated to allow alignment of an anatomically correct hand model developed by Atomedge to a 3D printed version of the computer graphic. For fiducial registration, the Vuforia Engine was added to test the alignment and spatial stability of the registered virtual object. The LMC and corresponding Orion SDK were combined with the HoloLens to explore markerless tracking.

The HoloLens has the tracking modules, the video camera modules, the central processing unit, and the display models built into one complete unit making it a suitable AR platform on which to explore the development of an AR HMD medical system. It ran the developed software application untethered for spatial mapping, virtual object computing, image processing, and rendering via the display module. All three of the developed AR HMD systems outperformed the required 30fps requirement for realistic visualisation. The fiducial marker tracking registration method performing the best out of the three proposed registration methods. Unfortunately, the registration performance, spatial alignment ability, and spatial stability of the three AR HMD systems would render all unsuitable as an intra-surgical guidance AR HMD medical system.

8.1 Improving the accuracy of registration

A recent project is the AR HMD medical system developed by Meulstee et al. (2019). Their system does not register the virtual to a real-world object, performing the converse instead; registering the real-world to the virtual. The virtual object is placed in the FOV of the user via the HoloLens and a tracked real-world object, with a collection of reflective spheres attached, is moved to where the virtual object is perceived.

An optical tracking system, similar to the Polaris optical tracking system, is used to identify the pose of the real-world object, concurrently. Fiducial markers attached to the HoloLens enable the optical tracking system to discern the transformation matrix between the real-world object and the HoloLens's FOV. In their validation, the captured positions of the real-world object were measured against the position specifications of the pre-guidance simulation. They reported a mean distance error of 2.3mm with a 0.5mm standard deviation between the planned location of the object and the resultant difference after placing the real-world object being tracked under AR navigation.

Adding a tracked stylus to correct the registration error identified between the virtual and real-world object may result in an optimal registration process. Making use of the tracked stylus and optical tracking system is one of the more common methods for integrating multimodal images of the patient on the 2D displays and the tracked instruments into a common coordinate system in IGS. However, the use of 2D displays does not utilise the enhanced visualisation capabilities of 3D AR views.

8.2 Improving the spatial capabilities (alignment and stability)

Although the registration performance of the three AR HMD systems showed the feasibility of the various registration methods, the size (>2mm) of the misalignment errors identified have made the developed AR HMD systems unsuitable for intra-surgical guidance.

Registration errors were identified during the assessment of all three of the AR HMD systems. Most notably, the spatial alignment errors due to the drift of the 3D virtual object as the user (clinician) moved around the real-world object (patient) in Jux3DModel and JuxL_Combo. As such, an exploration into different ways for increasing hologram stability is recommended.

The Microsoft Windows Dev centre recommended adding the SpatialAnchor Class to assist in hologram stability. The SpatialAnchor Class marks a virtual object in the virtual spatial map created as a point to calculate measurements from. From the MRTK SDK documentation it was understood that by adding the TapToPlace component to the FPS prefab, the SpatialAnchor Class would be assigned with to the FPS visualization to act as an anchor point (Figure 8.1). However, the spatial alignment results noted during the Jux3DModel and the JuxL_Combo application trials were notably worse than the spatial alignment results of the Frantz et al. (2018) control application. Thus enabling the SpatialAnchor class could also be assigned as a possible point of failure in the developed AR HMD systems and needs to be further explored.

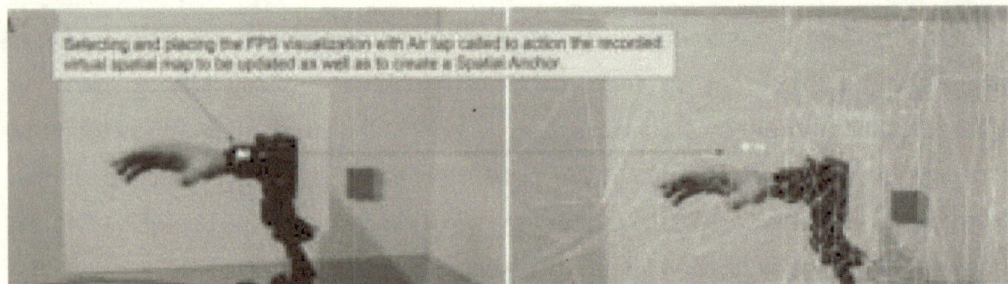

Figure 8.1: Placing the FPS virtual object to create a Spatial Anchor.

8.3 Conclusion

To improve registration, all three techniques could be combined into one single AR HMD medical system as none of the systems can be used in isolation. This is exemplified by the fact that the user perception of the visualisation from the stereoscopic rendering would require a form of user calibration for each clinician. All three of the AR HMD systems making use of the HoloLens underperformed the specifications of the required system. In its current form, the HoloLens could be considered as a device for exploring AR HMD medical systems for clinicians rather than a platform for building actual clinical applications. Seen as a prototyping device, the HoloLens becomes a powerful instrument to explore specific AR use cases. A secondary benefit of the HoloLens platform is as an accelerator for development in 3D medical visualisation, autonomous image processing, and development of user interfaces to aid clinicians.

8.4 Future work

As identified in chapter 3, the current form of the AR visualizations has mostly been static images which limit the functional understanding of anatomy such as joints. The markerless tracking system reported in this dissertation allows for AR visualization of patient movements viewed in real-time. To allow for an animation of the patient-specific bone geometries, a biomechanical model or "rig" of the patient's movements would have to be developed and combined with the virtual objects. The addition of real-time limb tracking to animate the juxtaposed AR visualization could possibly aid in understanding the complex properties of the anatomy in question during visualization, pre-surgical planning and post-operative review. Such a system could permit an understanding of the surgical site without additional radiological imaging. Qualitative and usability analysis of computer-mediated reality systems and AR visualizations was not part of the scope of work of this project and could be included in future work.

References

- Alam, F., Rahman, S.U., Ullah, S. & Gulati, K. 2018. Medical image registration in image guided surgery: Issues, challenges and research opportunities. *Biocybernetics and Biomedical Engineering*. 38(1):71–89. DOI: 10.1016/j.bbe.2017.10.001.
- Andress, S., Johnson, A., Unberath, M., Winkler, A.F., Yu, K., Fotouhi, J., Weidert, S., Osgood, G., et al. 2018. On-the-fly augmented reality for orthopedic surgery using a multimodal fiducial. *Journal of Medical Imaging*. 5(02):1. DOI: 10.1117/1.jmi.5.2.021209.
- Atrsaei, A., Salarieh, H. & Alasty, A. 2016. Human Arm Motion Tracking by Orientation-Based Fusion of Inertial Sensors and Kinect Using Unscented Kalman Filter. *Journal of Biomechanical Engineering*. 138(9):091005. DOI: 10.1115/1.4034170.
- Azimi, E., Qian, L., Navab, N. & Kazanzides, P. 2017. Alignment of the Virtual Scene to the Tracking Space of a Mixed Reality Head-Mounted Display. Available: http://arxiv.org/abs/1703.05834 [2019, January 02].
- Azuma, R.T. 1997. A Survey of Augmented Reality. Presence: Teleoperators and Virtual Environments. *Proceedings of the workshop for facial and bodily expressions for control and adaptation of games (ECAG 2008)*. 1(4):355–385. DOI: 10.1162/pres.1997.6.4.355.
- Backus, B.T., Dornbos, B.D., Tran, T.A., Blaha, J.B. & Gupta, M.Z. 2018. Use of virtual reality to assess and treat weakness in human stereoscopic vision. *IS and T International Symposium on Electronic Imaging Science and Technology*. 2018(4):1091–1096. DOI: 10.2352/ISSN.2470-1173.2018.04.SDA-109.
- Baltzer, H.L. & Moran, S.L. 2016. DOI: 10.1016/j.hcl.2016.07.003.
- Barfield, W. 2015. *Fundamentals of Wearable Computers and Augmented Reality*. W. Barfield, Ed. CRC Press. DOI: 10.1201/b18703.
- Barsom, E.Z., Graafland, M. & Schijven, M.P. 2016. Systematic review on the effectiveness of augmented reality applications in medical training. *Surgical Endoscopy and Other Interventional Techniques*. 30(10):4174–4183. DOI:

10.1007/s00464-016-4800-6.

- Beaulieu, A., Shepard, T. & Ellis, R. 2008. A process control system model for interactive image guided surgery. *2008 IEEE International Systems Conference Proceedings, SysCon 2008.* 70–77. DOI: 10.1109/SYSTEMS.2008.4518990.
- Beizer, B. & Wiley, J. 2005. *Black Box Testing: Techniques for Functional Testing of Software and Systems.* V. 13. Wiley. DOI: 10.1109/ms.1996.536464.
- Benford, S., Greenhalgh, C., Reynard, G., Brown, C. & Koleva, B. 1998. Understanding and Constructing Shared Spaces with Mixed-Reality Boundaries. *ACM Transactions on Computer-Human Interaction.* 5(3):185–223. DOI: 10.1145/292834.292836.
- Betts, J.G., Desaix, P., Johnson, E., Johnson, J.E., Koral, O., Kruse, D., Poe, B., Wise, J.A., et al. 2013. *Anatomy & Physiology.* Available: https://openstax.org/details/books/anatomy-and-physiology.
- Billinghurst, M., Clark, A. & Lee, G. 2014. A survey of augmented reality. *Foundations and Trends in Human-Computer Interaction.* 8(2–3):73–272. DOI: 10.1561/1100000049.
- Blum, T., Kleeberger, V., Bichlmeier, C. & Navab, N. 2012. Mirracle: An augmented reality magic mirror system for anatomy education. In *Proceedings - IEEE Virtual Reality.* IEEE. 115–116. DOI: 10.1109/VR.2012.6180909.
- Bork, F., Stratmann, L., Enssle, S., Eck, U., Navab, N., Waschke, J. & Kugelmann, D. 2019. The Benefits of an Augmented Reality Magic Mirror System for Integrated Radiology Teaching in Gross Anatomy. *Anatomical Sciences Education.* (February, 19):0–2. DOI: 10.1002/ase.1864.
- Bowen, W.T. & Slaven, E.M. 2014. Available: https://www.ebmedicine.net/media_library/files/1214 Hand Injuries(1).pdf [2018, April 25].
- Brouillette, D., Thivierge, G., Marchand, D. & Charland, J. 2012. Preparative study regarding the implementation of a muscular fatigue model in a virtual task simulator. *Work.* 41(SUPPL.1):2216–2225. DOI: 10.3233/WOR-2012-1024-2216.
- Butt, A.H., Rovini, E., Dolciotti, C., Bongioanni, P., De Petris, G. & Cavallo, F. 2017. Leap motion evaluation for assessment of upper limb motor skills in Parkinson's disease. In *IEEE International Conference on Rehabilitation*

Robotics. IEEE. 116–121. DOI: 10.1109/ICORR.2017.8009232.

- Carlsson, S. & Carlsson, E. 2013. "The situation and the uncertainty about the coming result scared me but interaction with the radiographers helped me through": A qualitative study on patients' experiences of magnetic resonance imaging examinations. *Journal of Clinical Nursing*. 22(21–22):3225–3234. DOI: 10.1111/jocn.12416.
- Carmigniani, J., Furht, B., Anisetti, M., Ceravolo, P., Damiani, E. & Ivkovic, M. 2011. Augmented reality technologies, systems and applications. *Multimedia Tools and Applications*. 51(1):341–377. DOI: 10.1007/s11042-010-0660-6.
- Carrino, F., Rizzotti, D., Gheorghe, C., Kabasu Bakajika, P., Francescotti-Paquier, F. & Mugellini, E. 2014. Augmented reality treatment for phantom limb pain. In *Lecture Notes in Computer Science (including subseries Lecture Notes in Artificial Intelligence and Lecture Notes in Bioinformatics)*. V. 8526 LNCS. Springer, Cham. 248–257. DOI: 10.1007/978-3-319-07464-1_23.
- Chen, L., Day, T.W., Tang, W. & John, N.W. 2017. Recent developments and future challenges in medical mixed reality. *Proceedings of the 2017 IEEE International Symposium on Mixed and Augmented Reality, ISMAR 2017*. (August, 3):123–135. DOI: 10.1109/ISMAR.2017.29.
- Chen, X., Xu, L., Wang, Y., Wang, H., Wang, F., Zeng, X., Wang, Q. & Egger, J. 2015. Development of a surgical navigation system based on augmented reality using an optical see-through head-mounted display. *Journal of Biomedical Informatics*. 55:124–131. DOI: 10.1016/j.jbi.2015.04.003.
- Citardi, M.J., Agbetoba, A., Bigcas, J.L. & Luong, A. 2016. Augmented reality for endoscopic sinus surgery with surgical navigation: A cadaver study. *International Forum of Allergy and Rhinology*. 6(5):523–528. DOI: 10.1002/alr.21702.
- Cosentino, F., John, N.W. & Vaarkamp, J. 2014. An overview of augmented and virtual reality applications in radiotherapy and future developments enabled by modern tablet devices. *Journal of Radiotherapy in Practice*. 13(3):350–364. DOI: 10.1017/S1460396913000277.
- Daponte, P., De Vito, L., Picariello, F. & Riccio, M. 2014. State of the art and future developments of the Augmented Reality for measurement applications. *Measurement*. 57:53–70. DOI: 10.1016/j.measurement.2014.07.009.

- Deebika, D. 2015. Augmented Reality advancement X-ray imaging medical reality scanning. *Biomedical and Pharmacology Journal*. 8(1):371–377. DOI: 10.13005/bpj/623.
- Dey, A., Billinghurst, M., Lindeman, R.W. & Swan, J.E. 2018. A Systematic Review of 10 Years of Augmented Reality Usability Studies: 2005 to 2014. *Frontiers in Robotics and AI*. 5:37. DOI: 10.3389/frobt.2018.00037.
- Diaz, C., Walker, M., Szafir, D.A. & Szafir, D. 2017. Designing for depth perceptions in augmented reality. In *Proceedings of the 2017 IEEE International Symposium on Mixed and Augmented Reality, ISMAR 2017*. IEEE. 111–122. DOI: 10.1109/ISMAR.2017.28.
- Douglas, D., Wilke, C., Gibson, J., Boone, J. & Wintermark, M. 2017. Augmented Reality: Advances in Diagnostic Imaging. *Multimodal Technologies and Interaction*. 1(4):29. DOI: 10.3390/mti1040029.
- Douglas, D.B., Venets, D., Wilke, C., Gibson, D., Liotta, L., Petricoin, E., Beck, B. & Douglas, R. 2018. Augmented Reality and Virtual Reality: Initial Successes in Diagnostic Radiology. In *State of the Art Virtual Reality and Augmented Reality Knowhow*. InTech. DOI: 10.5772/intechopen.74317.
- Duncan, S.F.M., Saracevic, C.E. & Kakinoki, R. 2013. Biomechanics of the hand. *Hand Clinics*. 29(4):483–492. DOI: 10.1016/j.hcl.2013.08.003.
- Eck, U., Stefan, P., Laga, H., Sandor, C., Fallavollita, P. & Navab, N. 2016. Exploring Visuo-Haptic augmented reality user interfaces for Stereo-tactic neurosurgery planning. In *Lecture Notes in Computer Science (including subseries Lecture Notes in Artificial Intelligence and Lecture Notes in Bioinformatics)*. V. 9805 LNCS. Springer, Cham. 208–220. DOI: 10.1007/978-3-319-43775-0_19.
- El-Gamal, F.E.Z.A., Elmogy, M. & Atwan, A. 2016. DOI: 10.1016/j.eij.2015.09.002.
- El-Hariri, H., Pandey, P., Hodgson, A.J. & Garbi, R. 2018. Augmented reality visualisation for orthopaedic surgical guidance with pre- and intra-operative multimodal image data fusion. *Healthcare Technology Letters*. 5(5):189–193. DOI: 10.1049/htl.2018.5061.
- Ferroli, P., Tringali, G., Acerbi, F., Schiariti, M., Broggi, M., Aquino, D. & Broggi, G. 2013. Advanced 3-dimensional planning in neurosurgery. *Neurosurgery*.

72(SUPPL. 1):A54–A62. DOI: 10.1227/NEU.0b013e3182748ee8.

- Frantz, T., Jansen, B., Duerinck, J. & Vandemeulebroucke, J. 2018. Augmenting microsoft's HoloLens with vuforia tracking for neuronavigation. *Healthcare Technology Letters*. 5(5):221–225. DOI: 10.1049/htl.2018.5079.
- Gabbard, J.L., Swan, J.E., Zedlitz, J. & Winchester, W.W. 2010. More than meets the eye: An engineering study to empirically examine the blending of real and virtual color spaces. In *2010 IEEE Virtual Reality Conference (VR)*. IEEE. 79–86. DOI: 10.1109/VR.2010.5444808.
- Gibby, J.T., Swenson, S.A., Cvetko, S., Rao, R. & Javan, R. 2019. Head-mounted display augmented reality to guide pedicle screw placement utilizing computed tomography. *International Journal of Computer Assisted Radiology and Surgery*. 14(3):525–535. DOI: 10.1007/s11548-018-1814-7.
- Green, J.B., Deveikas, C., Ranger, H.E., Draghetti, J.G., Groat, L.C., Schumer, E.D., Leslie, B.M., Draghetti, J.G., et al. 2016. Hand, Wrist, and Digit Injuries. In *Pathology and Intervention in Musculoskeletal Rehabilitation*. Elsevier. 344–435. DOI: 10.1016/B978-0-323-31072-7.00010-5.
- Hansen, C., Schostak, M., Detmer, F.J., Schindele, D. & Hettig, J. 2017. Virtual and Augmented Reality Systems for Renal Interventions: A Systematic Review. *IEEE Reviews in Biomedical Engineering*. 10:78–94. DOI: 10.1109/rbme.2017.2749527.
- Hugues, O., Fuchs, P. & Nannipieri, O. 2011. *Handbook of Augmented Reality*. V. 53. B. Furht, Ed. New York, NY: Springer New York. DOI: 10.1007/978-1-4614-0064-6.
- Kang, X., Azizian, M., Wilson, E., Wu, K., Martin, A.D., Kane, T.D., Peters, C.A., Cleary, K., et al. 2014. Stereoscopic augmented reality for laparoscopic surgery. *Surgical Endoscopy*. 28(7):2227–2235. DOI: 10.1007/s00464-014-3433-x.
- Katić, D., Spengler, P., Bodenstedt, S., Castrillon-Oberndorfer, G., Seeberger, R., Hoffmann, J., Dillmann, R. & Speidel, S. 2015. A system for context-aware intraoperative augmented reality in dental implant surgery. *International Journal of Computer Assisted Radiology and Surgery*. 10(1):101–108. DOI: 10.1007/s11548-014-1005-0.
- Kersten-Oertel, M., Jannin, P. & Collins, D.L. 2012. DVV: A taxonomy for mixed

reality visualization in image guided surgery. *IEEE Transactions on Visualization and Computer Graphics.* 18(2):332–352. DOI: 10.1109/TVCG.2011.50.

- Kersten-Oertel, M., Gerard, I.J., Drouin, S., Petrecca, K., Hall, J.A. & Collins, D.L. 2016. Towards augmented reality guided craniotomy planning in tumour resections. In *Lecture Notes in Computer Science (including subseries Lecture Notes in Artificial Intelligence and Lecture Notes in Bioinformatics).* V. 9805 LNCS. 163–174. DOI: 10.1007/978-3-319-43775-0_15.
- Khor, W.S., Baker, B., Amin, K., Chan, A., Patel, K. & Wong, J. 2016. Augmented and virtual reality in surgery-the digital surgical environment: Applications, limitations and legal pitfalls. *Annals of Translational Medicine.* 4(23):454–454. DOI: 10.21037/atm.2016.12.23.
- Kim, M.J., Park, J.M., Rhee, N., Je, S.M., Hong, S.H., Lee, Y.M., Chung, S.P. & Kim, S.H. 2012. Efficacy of VeinViewer in pediatric peripheral intravenous access: A randomized controlled trial. *European Journal of Pediatrics.* 171(7):1121–1125. DOI: 10.1007/s00431-012-1713-9.
- Kim, Y., Kim, H. & Kim, Y.O. 2017. Virtual reality and augmented reality in plastic surgery: A review. *Archives of Plastic Surgery.* 44(3):179–187. DOI: 10.5999/aps.2017.44.3.179.
- Köhler, N. 2017. Integration of a Leap Motion Controller with the HoloLens to enable improved gesture interactions. (December, 11). Available: https://aaltodoc.aalto.fi/handle/123456789/29268 [2018, April 11].
- Kolodzey, L., Grantcharov, P.D., Rivas, H., Schijven, M.P. & Grantcharov, T.P. 2017. Wearable technology in the operating room: A systematic review. *BMJ Innovations.* 3(1):55–63. DOI: 10.1136/bmjinnov-2016-000133.
- Kugelmann, D., Stratmann, L., Nühlen, N., Bork, F., Hoffmann, S., Samarbarksh, G., Pferschy, A., von der Heide, A.M., et al. 2018. An Augmented Reality magic mirror as additive teaching device for gross anatomy. *Annals of Anatomy.* 215:71–77. DOI: 10.1016/j.aanat.2017.09.011.
- Lachapelle, J.-M. 2014. The Hand: An Anatomoclinical Approach. In *Textbook of Hand Eczema.* Berlin, Heidelberg: Springer Berlin Heidelberg. 1–10. DOI: 10.1007/978-3-642-39546-8_1.
- Lee, K.-S. & Jung, M.-C. 2013. Biomechanics and Physical Ergonomics. In

Handbook of Loss Prevention Engineering. Weinheim, Germany: Wiley-VCH Verlag GmbH & Co. KGaA. 355–371. DOI: 10.1002/9783527650644.ch15.

- Lee, K.-S.S. & Jung, M.-C.C. 2015. *Ergonomic evaluation of biomechanical hand function*. V. 6. Elsevier. DOI: 10.1016/j.shaw.2014.09.002.
- Liszio, S. & Masuch, M. 2017. Virtual reality MRI: Playful reduction of children's anxiety in MRI exams. In *IDC 2017 - Proceedings of the 2017 ACM Conference on Interaction Design and Children*. New York, New York, USA: ACM Press. 127–136. DOI: 10.1145/3078072.3079713.
- Liu, L., Ecker, T.M., Siebenrock, K.A. & Zheng, G. 2016. Computer assisted planning, simulation and Navigation of periacetabular osteotomy. In *Lecture Notes in Computer Science (including subseries Lecture Notes in Artificial Intelligence and Lecture Notes in Bioinformatics)*. V. 9805 LNCS. Springer, Cham. 15–26. DOI: 10.1007/978-3-319-43775-0_2.
- Ma, L., Jiang, W., Zhang, B., Qu, X., Ning, G., Zhang, X. & Liao, H. 2019. Augmented reality surgical navigation with accurate CBCT-patient registration for dental implant placement. *Medical and Biological Engineering and Computing*. 57(1):47–57. DOI: 10.1007/s11517-018-1861-9.
- Mandalika, V.B.H., Chernoglazov, A.I., Billinghurst, M., Bartneck, C., Hurrell, M.A., Ruiter, N., Butler, A.P.H. & Butler, P.H. 2018. A Hybrid 2D/3D User Interface for Radiological Diagnosis. *Journal of Digital Imaging*. 31(1):56–73. DOI: 10.1007/s10278-017-0002-6.
- Mann, S., Furness, T., Yuan, Y., Iorio, J. & Wang, Z. 2018. All Reality: Virtual, Augmented, Mixed (X), Mediated (X,Y), and Multimediated Reality. *ArXiv*. abs/1804.0. Available: http://arxiv.org/abs/1804.08386 [2019, March 01].
- Meola, A., Cutolo, F., Carbone, M., Cagnazzo, F., Ferrari, M. & Ferrari, V. 2017. Augmented reality in neurosurgery: a systematic review. *Neurosurgical Review*. 40(4):537–548. DOI: 10.1007/s10143-016-0732-9.
- Meulstee, J.W., Nijsink, J., Schreurs, R., Verhamme, L.M., Xi, T., Delye, H.H.K., Borstlap, W.A. & Maal, T.J.J. 2019. Toward Holographic-Guided Surgery. *Surgical Innovation*. 26(1):86–94. DOI: 10.1177/1553350618799552.
- Mezger, U., Jendrewski, C. & Bartels, M. 2013. Navigation in surgery. *Langenbeck's Archives of Surgery*. 398(4):501–514. DOI: 10.1007/s00423-013-1059-4.

- Milgram, P. & Kishino, F. 1994. *Taxonomy of mixed reality visual displays*. Available: http://vered.rose.utoronto.ca/people/paul_dir/IEICE94/ieice.html [2018, November 29].
- Miller, J.A., Kwon, D.S., Dkeidek, A., Yew, M., Hisham Abdullah, A., Walz, M.K. & Perrier, N.D. 2012. Safe introduction of a new surgical technique: Remote telementoring for posterior retroperitoneoscopic adrenalectomy. *ANZ Journal of Surgery*. 82(11):813–816. DOI: 10.1111/j.1445-2197.2012.06188.x.
- Müller, M., Rassweiler, M.C., Klein, J., Seitel, A., Gondan, M., Baumhauer, M., Teber, D., Rassweiler, J.J., et al. 2013. Mobile augmented reality for computer-assisted percutaneous nephrolithotomy. *International Journal of Computer Assisted Radiology and Surgery*. 8(4):663–675. DOI: 10.1007/s11548-013-0828-4.
- Navab, N., Traub, J., Sielhorst, T., Feuerstein, M. & Bichlmeier, C. 2007. Action- and workflow-driven augmented reality for computer-aided medical procedures. *IEEE Computer Graphics and Applications*. 27(5):10–14. DOI: 10.1109/MCG.2007.117.
- Opriş, D., Pintea, S., García-Palacios, A., Botella, C., Szamosközi, Ş. & David, D. 2012. Virtual reality exposure therapy in anxiety disorders: A quantitative meta-analysis. *Depression and Anxiety*. 29(2):85–93. DOI: 10.1002/da.20910.
- Paul, P., Fleig, O. & Jannin, P. 2005. Augmented virtuality based on stereoscopic reconstruction in multimodal image-guided neurosurgery: Methods and performance evaluation. *IEEE Transactions on Medical Imaging*. 24(11):1500–1511. DOI: 10.1109/TMI.2005.857029.
- Pessaux, P., Diana, M., Soler, L., Piardi, T., Mutter, D. & Marescaux, J. 2014. Robotic duodenopancreatectomy assisted with augmented reality and real-time fluorescence guidance. *Surgical Endoscopy and Other Interventional Techniques*. 28(8):2493–2498. DOI: 10.1007/s00464-014-3465-2.
- Pourmand, A., Davis, S., Marchak, A., Whiteside, T. & Sikka, N. 2018. Virtual Reality as a Clinical Tool for Pain Management. *Current Pain and Headache Reports*. 22(8):53. DOI: 10.1007/s11916-018-0708-2.
- Pratt, P., Ives, M., Lawton, G., Simmons, J., Radev, N., Spyropoulou, L. & Amiras, D. 2018. Through the HoloLens™ looking glass: augmented reality for extremity reconstruction surgery using 3D vascular models with perforating

vessels. *European Radiology Experimental*. 2(1):2. DOI: 10.1186/s41747-017-0033-2.

- Preim, B. & Botha, C. 2013. Image-Guided Surgery and Augmented Reality. In *Visual Computing for Medicine*. Morgan Kaufmann. 625–663. DOI: 10.1016/b978-0-12-415873-3.00018-3.
- PTC Inc. 2018. Available: https://library.vuforia.com/articles/Training/Image-Target-Guide [2018, November 04].
- Qian, L., Barthel, A., Johnson, A., Osgood, G., Kazanzides, P., Navab, N. & Fuerst, B. 2017. Comparison of optical see-through head-mounted displays for surgical interventions with object-anchored 2D-display. *International journal of computer assisted radiology and surgery*. 12(6):901–910. DOI: 10.1007/s11548-017-1564-y.
- Rae, E., Lasso, A., Holden, M.S., Morin, E., Levy, R. & Fichtinger, G. 2018. Neurosurgical burr hole placement using the Microsoft HoloLens. In *Medical Imaging 2018: Image-Guided Procedures, Robotic Interventions, and Modeling*. V. 10576. R.J. Webster & B. Fei, Eds. SPIE. 20. DOI: 10.1117/12.2293680.
- Reitinger, B., Bornik, A., Beichel, R. & Schmalstieg, D. 2006. Liver surgery planning using virtual reality. *IEEE Computer Graphics and Applications*. 26(6):36–47. DOI: 10.1109/MCG.2006.131.
- Rodrigues, D.G., Jain, A., Rick, S.R., Liu, S., Suresh, P. & Weibel, N. 2017. Exploring Mixed Reality in specialized surgical environments. In *Conference on Human Factors in Computing Systems - Proceedings*. V. Part F127655. New York, New York, USA: ACM Press. 2591–2598. DOI: 10.1145/3027063.3053273.
- Schoob, A., Kundrat, D., Kahrs, L.A. & Ortmaier, T. 2017. Stereo vision-based tracking of soft tissue motion with application to online ablation control in laser microsurgery. *Medical Image Analysis*. 40:80–95. DOI: 10.1016/j.media.2017.06.004.
- Sheehan, S.E., Wortman, J.R. & Dyer, G.S.M. 2016. Traumatic Finger Injuries : What the Orthopedic Surgeon wants to know. *RadioGraphics*. 36(4):1106–1128. DOI: 10.1148/rg.2016150216.
- Shenai, M.B., Dillavou, M., Shum, C., Ross, D., Tubbs, R.S., Shih, A. & Guthrie,

B.L. 2011. Virtual interactive presence and augmented reality (VIPAR) for remote surgical assistance. *Neurosurgery*. 68(SUPPL. 1):ons200–ons207. DOI: 10.1227/NEU.0b013e3182077efd.

- Sherman, W.R. & B.Craig, A. 2018. Input: Interfacing the Participants with the Virtual World Understanding. In *Virtual Reality*. Second Edi ed. W.R. Sherman & A.B. Craig, Eds. (The Morgan Kaufmann Series in Computer Graphics). Boston: Morgan Kaufmann. 190–256. DOI: 10.1016/B978-0-12-800965-9.00004-0.
- Sielhorst, T., Feuerstein, M. & Navab, N. 2008. Advanced medical displays: A literature review of augmented reality. *IEEE/OSA Journal of Display Technology*. 4(4):451–467. DOI: 10.1109/JDT.2008.2001575.
- Soler, L., Nicolau, S., Pessaux, P., Mutter, D. & Marescaux, J. 2014. Real-time 3D image reconstruction guidance in liver resection surgery. *Hepatobiliary surgery and nutrition*. 3(2):73–81. DOI: 10.3978/j.issn.2304-3881.2014.02.03.
- Solovey, E.T., Okerlund, J., Hoef, C., Davis, J. & Shaer, O. 2015. Augmenting spatial skills with semi-immersive interactive desktop displays: Do immersion cues matter? In *ACM International Conference Proceeding Series*. V. 11. 53–60. DOI: 10.1145/2735711.2735797.
- Sutherland, J., Belec, J., Sheikh, A., Chepelev, L., Althobaity, W., Chow, B.J.W., Mitsouras, D., Christensen, A., et al. 2019. DOI: 10.1007/s10278-018-0122-7.
- Szeliski, R. 2011. Computer Vision: Algorithms and Applications. (Texts in Computer Science). London: Springer London. DOI: 10.1007/978-1-84882-935-0.
- Tosti, R. & Eberlin, K.R. 2018. DOI: 10.1016/j.hcl.2017.09.002.
- U.S. Food and Drug Administration. 2018. 510(k) Premarket Notification. 510:13–15. DOI: 10.1093/europace/eup008.
- Vassallo, R., Rankin, A., Chen, E.C.S. & Peters, T.M. 2017. Hologram stability evaluation for Microsoft HoloLens. In *Medical Imaging 2017: Image Perception, Observer Performance, and Technology Assessment*. V. 10136. M.A. Kupinski & R.M. Nishikawa, Eds. International Society for Optics and Photonics. 1013614. DOI: 10.1117/12.2255831.
- Vávra, P., Roman, J., Zonča, P., Ihnát, P., Němec, M., Kumar, J., Habib, N. &

El-Gendi, A. 2017. Recent Development of Augmented Reality in Surgery: A Review. *Journal of Healthcare Engineering*. 2017:1–9. DOI: 10.1155/2017/4574172.

- Voinea, A., Moldoveanu, A. & Moldoveanu, F. 2016. Bringing the augmented reality benefits to biomechanics study. In *Proceedings of the 2016 workshop on Multimodal Virtual and Augmented Reality - MVAR '16*. New York, New York, USA: ACM Press. 1–6. DOI: 10.1145/3001959.3001969.
- Wang, J., Shen, Y. & Yang, S. 2019. A practical marker-less image registration method for augmented reality oral and maxillofacial surgery. *International Journal of Computer Assisted Radiology and Surgery*. 14(5):763–773. DOI: 10.1007/s11548-019-01921-5.
- Wang, S., Parsons, M., Stone-McLean, J., Rogers, P., Boyd, S., Hoover, K., Meruvia-Pastor, O., Gong, M., et al. 2017. Augmented reality as a telemedicine platform for remote procedural training. *Sensors (Switzerland)*. 17(10):1–21. DOI: 10.3390/s17102294.
- Wu, M.L., Chien, J.C., Wu, C.T. & Lee, J. Der. 2018. An augmented reality system using improved-iterative closest point algorithm for on-patient medical image visualization. *Sensors (Switzerland)*. 18(8):2505. DOI: 10.3390/s18082505.
- Xie, T., Islam, M.M., Lumsden, A.B. & Kakadiaris, I.A. 2017. Holographic iRay: Exploring Augmentation for Medical Applications. In *Adjunct Proceedings of the 2017 IEEE International Symposium on Mixed and Augmented Reality, ISMAR-Adjunct 2017*. IEEE. 220–222. DOI: 10.1109/ISMAR-Adjunct.2017.73.
- Yoon, J.W., Chen, R.E., Kim, E.J., Akinduro, O.O., Kerezoudis, P., Han, P.K., Si, P., Freeman, W.D., et al. 2018. DOI: 10.1002/rcs.1914.
- Zhang, X., Wang, J., Wang, T., Ji, X., Shen, Y., Sun, Z. & Zhang, X. 2019. A markerless automatic deformable registration framework for augmented reality navigation of laparoscopy partial nephrectomy. *International Journal of Computer Assisted Radiology and Surgery*. (April, 23):1–10. DOI: 10.1007/s11548-019-01974-6.
- Zheng, G. & Nolte, L.P. 2015. Computer-Assisted Orthopedic Surgery: Current State and Future Perspective. *Frontiers in Surgery*. 2:66. DOI: 10.3389/fsurg.2015.00066.

- Zheng, G., Kowal, J., González Ballester, M.A., Caversaccio, M. & Nolte, L.P. 2007. Registration techniques for computer navigation. *Current Orthopaedics*. 21(3):170–179. DOI: 10.1016/j.cuor.2007.03.002.

www.ingramcontent.com/pod-product-compliance
Lightning Source LLC
LaVergne TN
LVHW041109150826
845673LV00007B/1982

* 9 7 8 3 3 8 4 2 2 1 1 2 4 *